Health after Chi[ld...]

An investigation of long term health problem[s] [beginnin]g
after childbirth in 11701 [women]

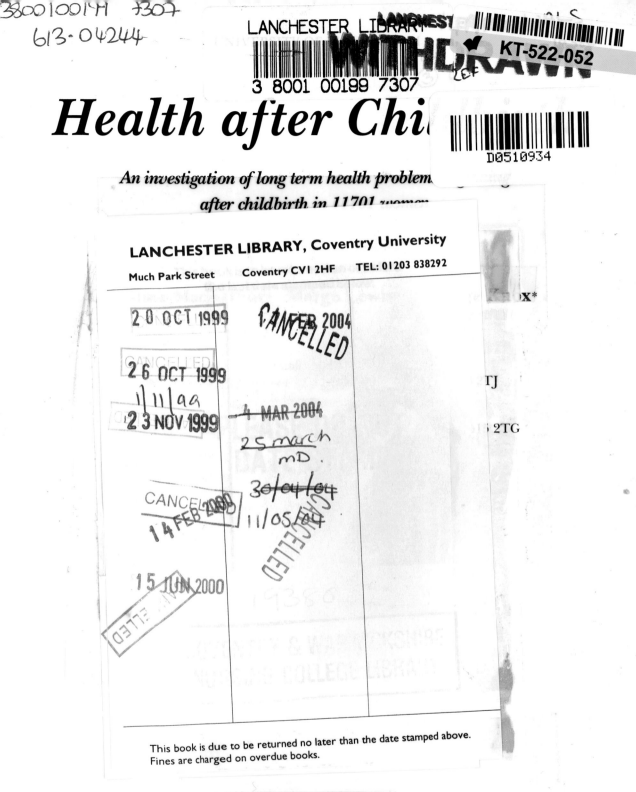

London : HMSO

Coventry University

Cover illustration by Jonathan Gooders

Acknowledgements

This study was supported by the Department of Health as part of a continuing programme of health services research within the Department of Public Health and Epidemiology. We thank the members of the Division of Obstetrics and Gynaecology of Birmingham Maternity Hospital for giving access to maternity records and the medical record officers for their practical help in answering numerous questions relating to the case notes. Many other members of the hospital staff also gave us advice on specific topics for which we are grateful. The 11701 women who took part in the study, providing the essential data on which the conclusions are founded deserve thanks too.

We record our thanks to Dr. J. Selwyn Crawford who was an instigator of the investigation and for whom we offer a tribute at the front of this volume.

Many members of the Department of Public Health and Epidemiology made essential contributions. Mrs. Pam Wills and Mrs. Sheila Allen typed countless drafts of this volume with accuracy, style and good humour. Mr. Robert Lancashire provided expert computer services. Ann Harvey, Sharon Murphy, Andrea Wright, Alison Green and Rachel Watkins gave assistance with numerous technical aspects of the research. Claire Wardroper also helped with much of the coding. Dr. Ken Cross and Mr. Tim Marshall supplied valuable statistical advice and Dr. Ciaran Woodman, Dr. Penny Blomfield and Dr. Heather Winter advised us on obstetric matters.

Finally, Catherine, Heather and William deserve a special mention for providing the first author with ample opportunity for participant observation.

Dr. Jeffrey Selwyn Crawford

M.B., Ch.B., M.D. (Illinois) F.F.A.R.C.S., F.R.C.O.G.

10.08.1922 – 16.08.1988

A tribute

Although not one of the authors of this book, Dr. Jeffrey Selwyn Crawford was involved in the original setting up of this study and he was party to the preliminary results, prior to his untimely death in 1988.

The feasibility of the study was also in large part due to Dr. Crawford's obsessive interest in data collection and clinical audit. He foresaw that it was essential to computerise anaesthetic records, a practice that was instituted at the Birmingham Maternity Hospital from an early stage, and which made the study possible.

Dr. Crawford was Consultant Anaesthetist at the Birmingham Maternity Hospital from 1968 to 1988 but even before this time had shown a unique dedication to the furtherance of obstetric anaesthesia. He was the author of 'Principles and Practice of Obstetric Anaesthesia': a founder member and inaugural President of the Obstetric Anaesthetists Association: and a prolific researcher and writer.

Reference to him locally as the 'Obstetric Monitor' was used as a term of respect and endearment: if occasionally of exasperation on the part of the obstetricians with whom he daily came in contact.

His knowledge of obstetric anaesthesia was encyclopaedic but, despite this and the worldwide esteem in which he was held, he was one of the most approachable of men; and his main concern was for the well-being, comfort and safety of all the mothers and their infants who passed through the doors of the Birmingham Maternity Hospital.

He would have been gladdened to see confirmation of his belief that childbirth is not such a 'natural' process after all and that it leads to an enormous amount of morbidity; but also saddened by the fact that it has received little recognition. He would have campaigned and researched energetically to discover means to reduce this post-partum morbidity: and harangued all around him (midwives, obstetricians, anaesthetists, etc.) to introduce any changes which might contribute towards its reduction.

Contents

Summary

Chapter 1 – Background to the Investigation

This investigation describes the types and measures the frequencies of health problems beginning after childbirth. It seeks out their potential determinants from among many different social, obstetric and anaesthetic factors. Chapter 1 describes how the study arose out of an initial enquiry concerning the possible long term consequences of epidural anaesthesia, and how it then developed to its final form. This was partly the result of technical necessities, but also reflected the evident scientific needs and the opportunities of the situation.

Chapter 2 – Purpose of the Study

This single page chapter sets out formally the main scientific objectives of the investigation.

Chapter 3 – Design of the Study

The design of the study was determined by four main considerations. The first was the initially formulated concern with long term rather than the more immediate sequelae of epidural anaesthesia. The second was a necessity to take simultaneous account of many different social, obstetric and anaesthetic factors which might also contribute to post-partum symptoms. A third was the requirement that the data on health problems should be obtained from a source independent of the maternity data. Finally, a prospective design – rather than a case-control design – was forced, because there was little evidence as to what the subsequent problems might be.

Contacting women after long intervals is difficult. A pilot study tested a postal method to see what proportion of women could be contacted, and what proportion of the contacted women would respond: in the event, an acceptable 80%. The eventual method of ascertainment was based on a postal questionnaire sent in January 1987 to all women delivering their most recent child in a Birmingham maternity hospital between 1978 and 1985. Of the 30,096 women who were sent questionnaires, 11701 returned them; a 'return' rate of only 39%. Like the pilot study much of the shortfall was due to migration, and among those who received the questionnaire, the 'response' rate was estimated to be 78%.

Chapter 4 – The Data Base

The maternity case-note data of the women who returned their questionnaires were compared with those who did not. This showed no differences in parity-distribution or in the obstetric or anaesthetic data, between the groups. However, there were some social differences, reflecting the greater residential mobility of young, single women, and women in ethnic minority groups. The 11701 returned questionnaires were linked to the maternity case-notes using the hospital registration number, to provide a data base consisting of combined records.

Chapter 5 – Analysis and Presentation of Data

The initial modes of analysis comprised the construction of frequency distributions and the measurement of simple associations between pairs of factors, particularly the health problems and their antecedents. These initial simple analyses were followed by multivariate discriminant analyses and multiway tabulations, in order to take simultaneous account of the complex inter-relationships between the many different factors, and to permit a search for the potential determinants of the different health problems.

Chapter 6 – Maternal, Obstetric and Anaesthetic Factors and their Relationships

The characteristics of the women, of their deliveries, and the relationships between these different factors are described in this chapter. The sample-data are compared with Birmingham birth-data, and with published national statistics. The main differences were that the sample contained more older women, fewer women in social class IV and V, fewer unmarried women and fewer first births. There were more Caesarean sections, more forceps deliveries and (probably) more epidurals. The effects of these variations upon extrapolations from the sample to the national population, are considered.

Chapter 7 – The Nature, Frequency and Durations of Health Problems

The overall results of the questionnaire data are described, and the choice of symptom 'acceptance-criteria' for inclusion in the main analysis is discussed. The frequencies of all health problems occurring at any time since the delivery, and of any duration – including those whose exact dates were not noted – are described first. We subsequently select only those occurring within three months of the delivery: and those lasting more than six weeks. Finally we limit 'acceptance' to those problems which had never been experienced before by the women. Any symptoms starting during pregnancy, or occurring at any time in the past, and those for which exact dates were not recorded, were all excluded. Even with these restrictions morbidity was widespread, with 47% of the women reporting at least one symptom. Although any symptom lasting more than six weeks was 'accepted', most had lasted much longer than this, and around two-thirds were still present at the time of our enquiry, 13 months to 9 years after the delivery.

Chapter 8 – Backache

Backache was a common health problem after delivery, with 1634 women (14% of the sample) reporting it as a newly occurring symptom, starting within three months of delivery, and lasting more than six weeks. Many backaches had become chronic and 65% of them had still not resolved at the time of our enquiry. There was a powerful association with epidural anaesthesia: 18.9% of women reported backache after an epidural compared with 10.5% after non epidural deliveries. This relationship was visible consistently in many different circumstances. The exception was after elective Caesarean Section. Differing pain tolerances did not seem to account for the epidural-association, nor did the excess of 'abnormal' deliveries associated with this procedure. Spinal anaesthesia and a long second stage of labour were additional independent predictors of backache, as was Asian ethnic group. We have suggested that the backache-producing mechanism is probably postural, occurring during labour in many women, but exacerbated by epidural anaesthesia through loss of muscle tone, inability to move, and inhibition of discomfort-feedback. Additional triggers in the post-partum environment (e.g. lifting, bending) are sometimes required before symptoms occur.

Chapter 9 – Frequent Headaches and Migraine

Frequent headaches, never previously experienced, starting within three months of delivery and persisting for more than six weeks, were reported by 3.6% of the sample; and 71% of these had lasted over a year. Migraine was less common, reported by 1.4% of the sample, with 85% of these cases lasting over a year. The two symptoms were found to have similar primary predictors and they jointly fell within one or other of two separate headache 'syndromes'. One was combined with backache, was closely associated with epidural anaesthesia and was more frequent among Asian women; these symptoms showed a striking pattern of onset-dates immediately after delivery. The second syndrome was unassociated with backache, and was unrelated to epidural but was more frequent in younger women, especially with more than one child. In these cases the symptoms started any time within the first three months, and some even afterwards. In the first combination we propose that the headaches can be regarded as the secondary symptoms of a posturally-related spinal axis syndrome. The second more probably represents a response to social stresses and pressures in the post-delivery environment.

Chapter 10 – Additional Musculo-Skeletal Symptoms

Additional musculo-skeletal symptoms (neckache; shoulderache; pain and weakness in the limbs and tingling in hands and feet) were individually infrequent, but as a group were reported by 8.2% of the sample. We looked for associations with the already postulated epidural-related spinal axis syndrome, and found that neckache and tingling in the hands/fingers appeared to be additional components of this symptom group. Our findings indicated the possible operation of two other sets of predictors. A striking excess of musculo-skeletal symptoms was reported by Asian women, especially pains and weakness in the limbs, where there was a four-fold excess. We have proposed that these symptoms might result from an underlying latent osteomalacia, exacerbated by the metabolic and physical stresses of pregnancy and delivery. Second, the combination of neckache, shoulderache and pain in the arms was associated with Caesarean section, especially with general anaesthesia. Only small numbers of women were affected here, but positioning of the neck to facilitate intubation suggests a plausible explanation. Through whatever of the various routes these different injuries might occur, they illustrate the extreme sensitivity to trauma of the skeletal/ligamentous system of the parturient woman.

Chapter 11 – Bladder Problems

Stress incontinence, starting as a new symptom within three months of delivery, and still unresolved, was reported by 10.6% of women delivering a first child. It was associated with long second-stage labours and big babies, and in some circumstances with forceps delivery. Increasing maternal age was another important predictor. Caesarean Sections resulted in lower symptom rates and even here the age-effect remained. Some previous investigators of stress incontinence have proposed that the major explanatory mechanisms of this symptom is damage to the innervation of the pelvic floor musculature. The factors associated with this damage corresponded in part with our own symptom predictors. However, our findings also provide evidence to suggest that the sphincter musculature may also be weakened through mechanisms other than a compressive neural injury and that the pathogenesis is more complex.

Urinary frequency was a less common bladder problem: it was reported as a new and unresolved symptom occurring after 4.9% of first births. Many cases of urinary frequency occurred jointly with stress incontinence, but for one third it occurred alone. Urinary frequency alone had no major delivery-related or maternal predictors and we have postulated this might have an infective rather than a directly traumatic component.

Chapter 12 – Haemorrhoids

Haemorrhoids starting within three months of delivery, and still unresolved, were reported by 5.3% of the women: 6.9% of primiparae. Unlike stress incontinence, the risk of new symptoms declined with increasing parity, suggesting a selective prior susceptibility, so that women who did not 'succumb' after their first delivery would be less susceptible after subsequent births. Deliveries with a greater degree of trauma – long second stage labour, forceps, heavier babies – resulted in higher rates of haemorrhoids, while a Caesarean section protected. These combined predictors produced variations in symptom rates ranging from 4.2% after Caesarean section, to 18% following a 2nd stage of three hours or more with a forceps delivery.

Chapter 13 – Depression, Anxiety and Extreme Tiredness

Depression and/or anxiety was reported as a new post-partum symptom lasting more than six weeks by 9.1% of the sample; and 12.2% reported extreme fatigue. These conditions showed less tendency to chronicity than most of the other symptoms: only 27% of the cases of depression and 39% of fatigue were still unresolved at the time of questioning.

A long first-stage labour was associated with depression and with fatigue, and a Caesarean section with depression, but only after a first birth. The obstetric associations did not suggest any of the direct physical mechanisms implicated for the musculo-skeletal or pelvic groups of symptoms. Post-partum haemorrhage, and inhalation analgesia for pain relief, were both related to fatigue: the first, through anaemia, the second needs investigating. However the main predictors of depression and fatigue were located within the domestic environment. This is compatible with numerous previous investigations on postnatal depression. Depression was more common among young mothers, and it was less common among Asians. Fatigue was more common among older mothers, and especially after a first birth. The unmarried state was highly predictive of depression and of fatigue, especially together, and especially for symptoms not yet resolved. Twins followed a similar pattern and so did a small baby. Breast feeding was also related to combined fatigue and depression, although only for complaints lasting less than one year.

Chapter 14 – Less Frequent Symptoms

Several less frequent symptoms were reported in response to specific questions, and others in response to an open question. Some of these infrequent symptoms, for example dental problems, indigestion, bowel problems, had been included as 'control' symptoms in order to detect general over-reporting after more 'invasive' procedures, especially epidurals, or sections. They helped us to confirm the validity of our findings in relation to these procedures. Other symptoms however showed associations with obstetric events. Epidurals were associated with dizziness or fainting: and a small proportion (0.5%) of women reported paraesthesias in lower parts of the body after epidural; this in response to the open enquiry. Buzzing in the ears, visual disturbances and dizziness/fainting were more frequent after general anaesthesia, with a combined relative risk of 1.36: this is difficult to explain. Finally, we noted that about 8% of the women with pregnancy-induced hypertension, reported raised blood pressure continuing for more than six weeks after the delivery, with half of these cases still unresolved. Further enquiries based on direct blood pressure measurement are required to confirm this.

Chapter 15 – Symptom-Clusters and 'Syndromes'

This chapter describes cross-associations between different symptoms. It shows that particular methodological technicalities, for example the exclusion of all inaccurately recorded symptoms, results in a degree of cross-correlation between the presence of the 'accepted' symptoms. It also indicates the possibility of neurotic or hyperchondriacal reporting in some women. But the main explanations of the major symptom clusters related to their common underlying mechanisms.

Chapter 16 – Synthesis

The main results of the investigation are summarised, the implications for the general population are calculated, and a range of technical issues are reviewed. The findings are then put together into a model etiological framework, based on three sets of potential symptom-determining factors, located in the mother's pre-delivery background, the delivery itself, and the post-partum environment.

Chapter 17 – Implications for Action

The final chapter presents the implications of the findings in terms of the suggested action. This is discussed at several different levels relating to fundamental research, preventive and therapeutic trials, and administrative rearrangements. They cover such issues as antenatal nutritional assessments in Asian women; the identification of circumstances pre-disposing to depression; the refinement of anaesthetic procedures; selective health education of women at high risk of bladder symptoms and haemorrhoids; post-partum assessments of haemoglobin levels; and more. Many require fundamental research followed by modified regimes of care accompanied by monitoring and evaluation.

Finally, and following confirmation of our findings, we recommend that consideration be given to replacing the standard six week postnatal follow-up by a progressive system of selective post-partum discharge, guided by a more adequate recognition of the full range of chronic post-childbirth morbidity as identified in this investigation.

A Note to Readers

This book has been written partly to cater for readers who are solely interested in particular symptoms, rather than in the results of the investigation as a whole. In order to meet their needs, and so that the chapters on particular symptoms (Chapters 8-14) can stand alone, certain materials are repeated in each of them. Readers interested in the full range of results should bear this in mind.

Chapter 1 – Background to the Investigation

This book describes the nature and measures the extent of health problems beginning for the first time following childbirth. It proceeds then to investigate their potential determinants. It seeks out the predictors of this ill health from among the social and demographic characteristics of the mother, the circumstances of her latest delivery, and the use of different obstetric and anaesthetic procedures.

This broad task developed out of an initial question posed by obstetric anaesthetists relating to one specific procedure: epidural anaesthesia. This procedure has been increasingly used over the last twenty years for pain relief during labour; and, more recently, as an alternative form of anaesthesia for Caesarean sections. At the Birmingham Maternity Hospital, where this enquiry was initiated, epidurals have been available routinely for pain relief since 1968 and all women who had an epidural were monitored daily whilst still in hospital to ascertain the nature of any side effects. By the time of this enquiry, 33,500 epidurals had been administered at the hospital and the extent and nature of the short-term side-effects had already been carefully assessed and documented. Much information had thus become available and had been reported, both from the Birmingham series and from elsewhere, concerning the immediate sequelae of the procedure (Crawford J.S. 1985a; 1985b; 1972: Ramanthan S. 1988). However, there had up to now been no opportunity to carry out a local study to test the possible existence of longer-term effects, and there appeared to be little or nothing on this subject in the medical literature. We therefore set out to repair this defect in our knowledge.

There were no prior indications that any long-term problems in fact existed, either on theoretical grounds, or from published anecdotal commentaries of patients or obstetricians. However, for a procedure administered as frequently as epidural anaesthesia we thought it necessary to establish positively, if such be the case, that the procedure was indeed free from long-term complications.

Broadening of the study design

While designing the study it became clear that there would be major methodological complexities both in collecting the data and in their analysis. As we tackled these problems and developed solutions, we found ourselves driven along a pathway of increasing data requirements and increasing scale. We began to understand why no similar survey had previously been reported.

The main design considerations were as follows:

1. Since no specific long-term effects of epidural anaesthesia had been reported in advance, or even formulated on theoretical grounds, it would be necessary to investigate a very wide variety of potential health problems if we were to be able to state with any confidence that there were no ill effects. Some of these problems might occur at quite low frequencies, and yet be important. It became clear that the investigation was going to involve large numbers of women.

2. Women who did not have an epidural during their delivery would of course have to be included in the study population in order to provide a proper comparison group. Many health problems following childbirth may occur irrespective of the particular procedures used, so conclusions relating to epidural anaesthesia would depend critically upon careful comparisons with controls.

3. Epidural anaesthesia is known to be more commonly used in particular obstetric circumstances (e.g. following induction of labour, in multiple pregnancy, with atypical fetal presentations, etc.) and for certain categories of women (e.g. primiparae). It is also more frequently associated with complicated deliveries (e.g. longer second stage labours, forceps deliveries, Caesarean sections). If post-partum health problems are also more frequent following these more difficult circumstances, this could result in a spurious statistical association between epidural anaesthesia and subsequent ill-health. Proper allowance for such 'confounding' variables requires simultaneous analysis of as wide a variety of obstetric and maternal factors as is possible. It also requires the participation of even larger numbers of women.

4. In constructing a health-enquiry schedule for the women, questions relating to different forms of pain relief would need to be included, to ensure that the respondents would not suppose that epidural anaesthasia was a particular focus of the investigation. Responses from those women who had (or did not have) an epidural, could thus be freed as much as possible from conscious or attitudinal bias.

The final plan

It had become clear that to investigate the possible longer-term effects of epidural anaesthesia alone would necessitate an enquiry of considerable scale and complexity. If we had to embark upon so large and so complex a study, would it not be more economical, and statistically more powerful, to broaden the objectives? Should we not enquire simultaneously into other potential symptom-predicting factors, both maternal and obstetric, rather than treat them only as 'confounder' variables in an investigation limited to the long-term effects of epidurals?

The wider objective in turn demanded that we enquire more broadly into the nature of the women's post-partum health problems. However, it was foreseen that this added range of questioning would bring some technical advantages. There was a much reduced danger of biased responses from women who might read into some questions, the connections which we originally had in mind. In addition, questions pursuing the potential consequences of one procedure, would serve as 'dummy'-information, and as a negative check, for investigating another procedure.

For all these reasons we decided to undertake a more general investigation of the prevalence of longer-term health problems following childbirth: and their associations with the full recorded range of social, obstetric and anaesthetic circumstances and procedures. The medical literature is sparse on many of these points so these broader objectives would provide a valuable addition to our knowledge on post-partum health, as well as encompassing more effectively the questions originally raised concerning the long-term effects of epidural anaesthesia.

There was also a certain novelty in asking women how they had fared, overall, in the years following a delivery. As we reviewed the literature it became clear that no-one had ever thought of asking them before!

Chapter 2 – Purpose of the Study

The purpose of the study as eventually formulated, incorporated four main scientific objectives. These were:

1. To ascertain the types and measure the frequencies and durations of long-term health problems occurring after childbirth, through direct enquiry, in a reasonably representative sample of women in Britain.

2. To describe the social and demographic characteristics of the women in the sample as recorded in the maternity case-notes; to describe the events of the delivery, and the types and frequencies of the obstetric and anaesthetic procedures which they experienced, using the same source; to measure the inter-relationships between all these events, characteristics and procedures.

3. To investigate the associations between the later health problems as reported directly by the women (1 above): and their recorded social and demographic characteristics and the obstetric and anaesthetic processes and procedures which they received (2 above).

4. To dissect the complex inter-relationships between all these factors and the reported health problems in order to separate those associations which might be counted as primary, from those which were more likely to be secondary. We would then try to identify the particular social, obstetric or anaesthetic predictors and potential determinants of the various health problems reported.

Chapter 3 – Design of the Study

The objectives as formulated, and the scientific criteria necessary for identifying the potential determinants of health outcomes, demanded:

a. **A prospective design:** that is, we first had to identify women with different levels and different types of exposure to risk, and then follow them up to see what health problems they had experienced. This approach was imposed by the absence of well-founded prior hypotheses regarding the causes of particular health problems on which a retrospective case-control design could have been based.

b. **Large numbers:** our initial estimates, based on mock analyses, were that we needed a sample of about 10,000 women.

c: **Long-term follow-up:** Routine postnatal examinations at six weeks have elicited a basic knowledge of only short-term health problems following delivery. It is in the area of long-term problems that our knowledge is especially deficient.

Follow-up

The obstetric and anaesthetic data, and the basic social and demographic characteristics of the women, were available from the full computer-coded maternity case-notes. In order to obtain the follow-up data on health problems however, a postal questionnaire was the only practical means of collecting the necessary material from so many women, after intervals extending to nine years after delivery. This choice of method can be open to criticism on several grounds. Sometimes it attracts a low response rate, with the parallel risk of selection-bias and a resulting non-representative sample. In addition, the range and detail of the questions that can be asked using this method is limited, and there is always a risk that questions can be misunderstood. However, it has been shown that if participants are interested in the topic and if the questionnaire is kept short and clear, it is possible to elicit a good numerical response (MacArthur and Wakefield 1978); and Cartwright (1987) has recently shown that well-designed postal questionnaires proved a useful and effective data collection method in studying aspects of maternity services and childbirth in the UK. Postal questionnaires produced a good response as well as a high level of congruence between the mothers' answers to questions and the medical records (Martin 1987).

The design of the questionnaire to be sent to the women was therefore crucial. For this reason, and also to elicit the proportions of women still traceable at the latest address recorded in the hospital notes, we carried out a pilot survey.

Pilot study

The requirements for such large numbers, the need to study long-term health problems, and the necessity to specify the most recent birth, effectively defined the population from which enrolment could be invited. The sample had to be drawn from women who had delivered over a substantial period prior to the time of the enquiry. This raised a practical problem. Over so many intervening years we would expect some women to have moved house, so that many of the addresses in the maternity case-notes would be out of date. It was important to discover how many had moved, since this proportion of the population would probably not receive their questionnaire.

It was also necessary, for the purposes of assessing potential bias, to measure both the special characteristics of those who had moved, and the response rate among women who did in fact receive the questionnaire. If we obtained a low overall return rate, we needed to know whether this was mainly because the women had moved and had not received the questionnaire, or whether many of them had declined to complete and return it. If the latter, then we would have to assume that there could be significant biases of measured morbidity because women who had health problems, especially those which were persistent or severe, might be more motivated to take part in the study and return their questionnaire. If the former, then the problem would be less serious and the biases would be largely limited to the selective social circumstances of migration or non-migration. The primary objectives of the pilot study were to ascertain the proportion of questionnaires that would be returned: to distinguish between women who received the questionnaire and failed to reply, and women who never received it: and to assess the level at which individual questions were understood, and the quality of response.

The pilot study consisted of 250 deliveries. Of the 250 questionnaires sent, 88 (35%) were returned completed. Addresses of the remaining 162 were checked in Electoral Registers and with the Post Office, showing that only 22 of these women still seemed to reside at the address obtained from the maternity case-notes. These data gave us the answers to our first two questions. We could estimate that at least 56% of the sample (140) had moved from the address given in the hospital notes; whilst of 110 women still living at the same address, 80% (88) had returned their questionnaires completed. We could distinguish technically between a return rate of 35%: and a response rate of 80%. The first of these presents a logistical problem of obtaining adequate numbers: but the second is reassuring in that it excludes the possibility of gross outcome-related bias. We were also able to show, within the uncertainties of these limited numbers, that there were no gross social or obstetric selective biases among the group who returned their questionnaire forms, compared with the non-returners.

The other main objective of the pilot study was to assess the quality of the responses to the questions given on the questionnaire and, as far as possible, to see whether they had been well understood. The questions had been developed after several pre-pilot discussions with small groups of mothers. Our assessments after piloting were based chiefly upon a careful reading and cross-referencing of the responses. The questions on the pilot survey schedule seemed indeed to have been understood by the respondents. In addition we were able to check the accuracy of the women's recall for questions which could be compared with similar items of information recorded in the maternity case-notes. In fact most of these responses corresponded well with information already recorded in the obstetric records. This last conclusion was re-confirmed in the main survey, and the results will be described in more detail in a later chapter.

Given that only about a third of the questionnaires dispatched would be returned completed, and because we required about 10,000 participants, around 30,000 would have to be sent. In an attempt to reduce these numbers, we sought assistance from the local Family Practitioner Committee (FPC), to trace the new addresses of those women who had moved. We ascertained that their recently installed computer register was sufficiently accurate in these respects to make the exercise worthwhile. However, the Local Medical Committee then refused to give its approval for the systematic use of the register for the full survey. The FPC felt that it had to comply with its advice and the approach was thus barred to us.

We therefore decided to adopt the same method of contact for the main study as we had tested in the pilot study. The initial pilot findings had shown that a large scale postal questionnaire approach was feasible in this situation and likely to be productive.

Main study

The return rates from the pilot study indicated that in order to obtain the necessary 10,000 post-partum respondents we would have to send out around 30,000 questionnaires. We had ascertained that between 1978 and 1985, 30,096 women (excluding maternal and perinatal deaths) had delivered at least one baby at the maternity hospital used for the study. This was a convenient number for our purposes. The particular delivery years of 1978 to 1985 were chosen because the case-note information was recorded and stored on the hospital computer using a consistent format for the whole of the eight year period. Prior to 1978, the information in the maternity case-notes differed both in its content and in its format.

We excluded from the population all maternal and perinatal deaths, the former for obvious reasons, the latter because of the risk of causing unnecessary distress to the mother. The objectives of the study were such that the exclusion of perinatal deaths was unlikely to cause serious bias or loss of information. We could not however exclude subsequent child or maternal deaths unless there was a record of the death, as occasionally there was, in the maternity case-notes.

The population of 30,096 women were sent questionnaires in January 1987 together with a printed pre-paid return envelope. Women were asked to complete the questionnaire in relation to the delivery of their most recent child, the date of which was specified both on the questionnaire and in the accompanying covering letter (see Appendix 1). Of the 30,096 women, 11,701 completed and returned the questionnaires within 20 weeks, although most were return within the first 2 or 3 weeks. This 39% return rate was rather greater than in the pilot study. A further 45 questionnaires were returned too late to be included in the analysis, some of them up to two years later. Ten questionnaires were returned with accompanying letters saying that the woman had since died; four women wrote back refusing to take part in the study; and two questionnaires were discarded as unintelligible. There were also ten questionnaires that had been completed by the wrong women. Even though no names were attached to the returned questionnaires, these errors could be detected using the baby's date of birth. These ten women had all delivered babies at the study hospital and at the time of the enquiry must have been residing at an address formerly occupied by a woman in our sample. Some presumable failed to receive questionnaires directed to their previous address.

A repeat check of a 5% sample of non-returners was made in the same manner as for the pilot study. Through combining those which had been returned by the post office as 'moved away' and the results of another electoral-register scan, we confirmed that the majority of non-returners (82%) were no longer living at the address taken from the case-notes. We estimated that of the women who had not moved house and who presumably had received a questionnaire, 78% had completed and returned it.

Chapter 4 – The Data Base

The data for the study came from two separate sources. The data on the basic social and demographic characteristics of the mother and the obstetric and anaesthetic factors were obtained from computer-coded hospital case-notes. The information concerning subsequent health problems was obtained from the postal questionnaires returned by the women. Some items of data were available from both sources.

Maternity case-note data

Full maternity case-notes were available in computerised form for all the women in the study. The main items of information obtained from this source were: parity; maternal age at booking; marital status; social class; ethnic group; maternal height; presence or absence of antenatal complications (hypertension and ante-partum haemorrhage); type of onset of labour (spontaneous, induced); single or multiple birth; durations of first and second stage labour; fetal presentation (occipito-anterior, breech, etc); mode of delivery (Caesarean, vaginal unassisted, forceps); perineal complications (episiotomy, lacerations); post-partum haemorrhage; all types of pain relief and anaesthesia administered; gestation at delivery; the birthweight, head circumference, length and sex of the infant; admission to special care; type of infant feeding on discharge. These same case-note data were also available for those women who had not returned their questionnaires.

Questionnaire data

The postal questionnaire was kept very short – just one sheet of A4 paper printed on both sides – in order to ensure a high response from those women who received it. The first side requested factual information about the date and place of birth and the type of pain relief for each of the woman's deliveries as well as whether any had been by Caesarean section. The next questions elicited opinions about the effectiveness of all types of pain relief experienced during the index delivery. Lastly the women were asked about any major illnesses or operations they had had since that delivery. The date of the index delivery was clearly specified on the first side of the questionnaire. The second side of the questionnaire gave a list of 25 specific health problems or symptoms. For each health problem the woman was asked whether she had had it since the birth of the 'index' baby. Where the answer was 'Yes', she was also asked (1) whether she had ever had this particular problem or symptom before the birth; (2) how long after the birth had the symptom occurred; (3) how long after the birth it had ceased (or was continuing); (4) whether she had been to the doctor about it;

TABLE 4.1

Comparison of 'Returners' and 'Non-Returners'

	'Returners' (11701) No. (%)	'Non-returners' (19384) No. (%)
Primiparae	4185 (36)	6683 (36)
Under 25 years	2625 (22)	7078 (39)
25 – 29	4225 (36)	6170 (34)
30 or more	4851 (41)	5136 (28)
Married	10525 (90)	15107 (82)
Social class I, II	2882 (25)	3316 (18)
III, IV, V	7050 (60)	9971 (54)
Unclassified	1769 (15)	5097 (28)
Caucasian	10135 (87)	13864 (75)
Asian	530 (5)	1836 (10)
Afro-Caribbean	388 (3)	1108 (6)
Multiple pregnancy	169 (1)	244 (1)
Occipito-anterior fetal presentation	10265 (88)	16234 (88)
Induced labour	1437 (12)	2062 (11)
Duration of labour		
First stage under 6 hours	2195 (19)	3582 (20)
Second stage 1 hour or more	2798 (24)	3769 (21)
Forceps – straight	1858 (16)	2690 (15)
rotational	443 (4)	667 (4)
Elective section	770 (7)	997 (5)
Emergency section	1145 (10)	1672 (9)
Episiotomy	5112 (44)	8315 (45)
Laceration	2887 (25)	3825 (21)
Epidural anaesthesia	4766 (41)	6843 (37)
Pre-term gestation	800 (7)	1332 (7)
Birthweight 2500 grams or less	767 (7)	1382 (8)

and (5) what treatment, if any, she had had. In addition to these specific health problems there was one 'open-category' question, in which the woman was asked to identify any other problems she had experienced, with answers in the same format. A copy of the questionnaire and the covering letter is supplied in Appendix 1.

Combined data base

The hospital registration number for every woman was attached to the questionnaire sheet before it was sent out. Returned questionnaires could thus be entered to a computer file and subsequently linked using this number, to the original maternity case-note record for each woman. This meant that the names of the women were used only for addressing envelopes. Participants' names were not shown on the questionnaire forms, nor on the final data base, thus ensuring that the personal confidentiality of the survey data was fully protected. The record linking process was carried out by computer for all the 11,701 women who returned their questionnaires and the resulting combined maternity case-note and questionnaire material for these women comprised the data base on which the main analyses were carried out.

Comparison of returners and non-returners

In order to confirm that our method of obtaining the population had indeed provided us with an unbiased sample, it was important to examine the degree to which the respondents represented the total population which had been approached. Case-note information was obtained for all but 11 of the 19,395 women who did not return their questionnaires. Included with the non-returners were those women who had died in the intervening years (10), refused to answer (4), whose questionnaires were unintelligible (2), or returned too late (45), or completed by the wrong women (10). A comparison between the two groups is given in Table 4.1.

There were several socio-demographic differences between the 'returner' and 'non-returner' groups. More of the non-returners were unmarried; fewer were from social classes I and II and more were 'unclassified' for social class, mainly because they were single. More were under 25 years of age and fewer were aged 30 years or more. These maternal factors were themselves inter-related and the high estimated response rate among women who had actually received their questionnaires leads us to summarise differences between the groups in the terms that the younger, single, lower social class women had moved their residences more often. There were no differences between the 'returners' and 'non-returners' with respect to parity; 36% of the women in each group had delivered their first baby.

In addition there were significantly more Asian and Afro-Caribbean women among the non-returners. Some Asian women were probably unable to complete and return the questionnaires because of language difficulties. It is also likely that there are differences in the geographical mobility of recent immigrant groups. Each of these factors would result in fewer questionnaires being returned from these ethnic groups.

The essential question is whether differences in the social characteristics of the women who were not included in the study-sample, compared with those who were, could have influenced our measures of the frequencies of long-term health problems. The literature on the health of disadvantaged groups, including young, single, lower social class and 'ethnic-minority' women might lead us to expect that the non-returners would have had **more** health problems than the returners. Selective exclusion of 'disadvantaged' women through 'non-returning' might therefore lead to a **lower** apparent incidence of health problems within the study sample, compared with the population from which it was drawn.

However, the factors most directly relevant to the objectives of this study were the obstetric and anaesthetic circumstances, procedures and events. In these respects the returners and non-returners were virtually identical. If any of these obstetric or anaesthetic factors were found to be associated with particular health problems, then the exclusion of the non-returners would have made little difference to the results of the study.

The extent to which the study sample could be regarded as representative of the general population of parturient women in this country and in Birmingham as a whole, as opposed to the particular hospital, is described later in Chapter 6.

Reliability of data

We considered the reliability of the data obtained from the maternity case notes, and from the questionnaires. Problems relating to the two sources are quite different but both are important in assessing the accuracy of the study data. We also examined the concordances of data items obtained from both sources.

Maternity case note data

We cannot expect every item of information recorded in any hospital case notes to be totally accurate and random errors will always occur. Although great care, and numerous validity tests, are used in this particular hospital, there will inevitably be some errors in transferring the data to the computer. There were three potential sources of error corresponding with the three stages of the process: information was first handwritten into the case notes: this was next coded on to a coding sheet for computer entry: and thirdly the coded data was entered by keyboard to the computer. The data recording and data entry system now used by the hospital is more sophisticated, providing less scope for error, but at the time of these 1978-85 deliveries the earlier three-stage process of data recording was still in use.

In addition to random errors there was direct evidence of process-errors in that some items of information recorded twice in different connections did not match. The problems chiefly arose from ambiguous rules of definition. In most cases the numbers involved were very small; those involving larger numbers are described below.

Marital Status had a category for 'Single Women' and 908 were thus coded. The variable, **Social Class** was based on the occupation group of the woman's husband and included the category 'Single', since this group could not be classified in the same manner. Here, only 822 women were coded as single. Occasionally, especially for young single women still living with parents, the occupation of the woman's father was used for classifying social class. For the purposes of analyses we have used 'Single' as categorised under **Marital Status.**

Onset of Labour includes a code for 'Elective Caesarean Section', used for women who had a planned section with no onset of labour; 975 women were given this code. In a subsequent case note variable, **Type of Delivery** however, 770 women were coded as having an 'Elective Caesarean Section'. The 205 cases which did not match were coded here (in all but 5) as 'Emergency Caesarean Section'. Sometimes, for example where there is pre-eclampsia or fetal distress, a section will be completed before the onset of labour, but it would be coded as an emergency section because it was not pre-arranged. We have assumed that the coding under **Type of Delivery** was the correct one.

There were also some difficulties involved in interpreting combinations of items recorded under separate variables. For example in order to identify women delivered by Caesarean Section under epidural anaesthesia, we would have to use two separate items of information: the code for **Type of Delivery,** where those women having a section would be itemised: and the code for **Type of Anaesthesia** where epidural anaesthesia was specified. But some women so identified might first have had an epidural for pain relief, and a section later under general anaesthesia. To compile the group who had a section under epidural we had to look further at whether or not the women had had general anaesthesia as well. If so we have assumed that the section was itself carried out under general and not epidural anaesthesia. However, there may be one or two women who had the section under epidural, but who had a general anaesthetic after the delivery, for some other reason.

Questionnaire data

The accuracy of the reports returned by the responding women, and their understanding of the questions put to them, were assessed in two ways. First, we compared those items of information which were duplicated in both data sources. Second, we examined the women's recall of information by comparing their reports from more distant and more recent deliveries.

Duplicated information

Two specific items included in the questionnaire could be compared objectively with case-note material. The women were asked whether the index delivery had been a Caesarean section, and whether they had had epidural anaesthesia.

Caesarean section: The case-notes recorded that 1,915 of the 11701 respondents had a Caesarean section; and all but 38 (2%) of them also reported it on the questionnaire for the 'index' baby. Of the 9786 women whose case-notes did not record a section, 35 (0.35%), all multiparae, reported on the questionnaire that they had had one. Both of these 'errors' probably resulted from the women having become confused as to **which** baby was delivered by section. The low overall discrepancy rate, about 0.6%, indicates a very high accuracy of recall and a high level of attention to and understanding of the questions posed.

Epidural anaesthesia: In the maternity case-note 4766 of the 11701 respondents were recorded as having had epidural anaesthesia; all but 111 (1.6%) of these women confirmed this in the questionnaire. Of the 6935 women whose case-notes did not record an epidural, 351 (7.4%) said in the questionnaire that they had one. The overall discrepancy rate, at 3.9%, was higher than for Caesarean section.

However, 107 of the 351 women who gave a 'false-positive' report were recorded in the case-notes as having had spinal anaesthesia. Part of the problem was that they failed to discriminate between the two procedures. The distinction between them is a technical one, not clearly evident from the woman's point of view, so the confusion is scarcely surprising. If we allow for this, excluding the spinal anaesthesias, we obtain an overall discrepancy rate of 3.0% for the epidurals. Again, some women may have had an epidural for another child and failed after this interval of time, to remember exactly which one it was. In addition, for some women, an epidural may have been requested and commenced but abandoned in the very early stages, and not recorded as such in the case-notes.

Accuracy of distant recall

We might expect that health problems associated with deliveries occurring several years previously would be recalled less frequently and less accurately than those which had occurred more recently. Some of the women in this study had delivered their babies in 1978, nine years before the questionnaires were sent (January 1987). The most recent deliveries, on the other hand, had occurred only thirteen months before. A women who has experienced a symptom several years previously, even if it lasted for some months, is a priori less likely to recall it with the same degree of accuracy, if at all, than a woman who has delivered her baby more recently. We therefore compared the proportions of women reporting different health problems, and those with inadequately dated symptoms, according to the number of years that had elapsed since the delivery.

We found that the proportion of women who reported one or more symptoms as occurring some time after delivery but could not provide accurate dating, did increase with the duration of the intervening period: 36% for women delivering in 1978-79 and 24% for the 1984-85 deliveries. All inadequately dated symptoms, many of which would probably anyway have beeen short-term or occurring months or years after delivery, were excluded from our analyses (See Chapter 7).

We found too that the proportions of women reporting different symptoms increased, as the recall interval decreased. For example, 8.1% of the women who had delivered in 1978 and 1979 reported lower backache occurring for the first time in their lives, within three months of delivery and lasting longer than six weeks. For 1980 and 1981 deliveries, the proportion was 9.6%; for 1982 and 1983 deliveries, 10.3%; and for 1984 and 1985 deliveries, 12.4%. This pattern was not limited to backache: the same trend was evident for most of the symptoms examined. It is of course possible that there were genuine temporal changes, but the variations were systematic, and almost certainly resulted from recall-selection. This means that the true frequencies of most post-partum health problems are probably somewhat greater than appears from long-term retrospective recall. We discuss this in more detail in Chapter 7.

Acceptability

Our main conclusions regarding the data base were: (1) The maternity case-notes confirmed the accuracy of those questionnaire-based items with which they could be compared; (2) The reports of subsequent health problems, although based upon self perception appeared to provide meaningful statements of the ill health which these women subsequently suffered: (3) The response rate from women receiving a questionnaire was high, and no significant overall bias resulted from the exclusion of those who had not returned a questionnaire: (4) If there was an overall problem of symptom ascertainment, it was that the reporting method underestimated the true number of health problems.

Chapter 5 – Analysis and Presentation of Data

Copies of the full computer-coded maternity case-notes were transferred to magnetic tape and thence to the University main-frame computer. This primary case-note file served to identify the survey population, and from it were generated the labels for the questionnaire and also the addresses for the envelopes. The labels noted the date of birth of the index child and the mother's maternity hospital registration number in order to effect linkage of each woman's questionnaire and case-note data. The questionnaire data, when returned by the women, were entered first to micro-computer magnetic storage where they were checked and validated. These questionnaire data files were subsequently transferred 'on-line' to the main-frame computer and linked with the primary case-note file. This then provided a single record for each respondent containing both her questionnaire data and complete maternity case-note information. The analyses of the data were carried out using the Statistical Package for Social Scientists (SPSSX).

Methods of analyses

The analyses, and the presentations of data offered in this report are of four main types, namely (1) frequency distributions of single variables; (2) associations between different pairs of variables; (3) multivariate analyses, and (4) multi-way tabulations of two or more symptom-predictors against their presumed outcomes.

Frequency distributions

These were compiled to show the numbers and proportions of women who reported different health problems, and to display their onsets and durations. Frequency distributions of the numbers of women according to their social, demographic, obstetric and anaesthetic characteristics were compiled in a similar manner.

Associations between characteristics

Associations between pairs of factors were assembled at each of three levels. First, each of the socio-demographic, obstetric and anaesthetic factors was set out against each of the others. Next, each of these maternal and obstetric factors was related to each of the health problems. Since most of these factors were recorded in categorical format, the main form of presentation is the 2 × 2 or 2 ×

K Tables and the main test of statistical significance used for these was the chi-squared test of association, incorporating Yates' correction where relevant. If the item was represented as a continuous variable, for example maternal age, the t-test was used. In general, only tabulations indicating associations returning 5% and 1% levels of statistical significance are presented. Associations not reaching these levels of statistical significance have not generally been shown in this report. Finally, each of the health problems was related to each of the others.

Multivariate analysis

This was the essential analytical tool in this study. It was used in order to differentiate primary from secondary associations with a view to identifying potential causal relationships between the maternal and obstetric characteristics on the one hand, and the subsequent health problems, on the other.

The overall results revealed a complex pattern of associations between the many maternal, obstetric and anaesthetic factors and it was this which necessitated their simultaneous analyses in groups. An example will make this clearer. Forceps delivery is statistically associated with a prolonged second stage of labour, so that if **either** forceps **or** a prolonged second stage caused an increased risk of subsequent stress incontinence (say), a simple statistical association would appear for both. Having detected two such associations, we would then wish to know which could be regarded as primary, independent of the other and therefore a potential determinant, and which of them might only be 'secondary'. In addition, each of these factors might be related to the age of the mother, parity, type of pain relief, size of the infant, and so on. Multivariate analysis must be used in these complex situations to ascertain which particular maternal, obstetric or anaesthetic factors remained independently associated with a given health problem, after adjusting for the effects of all other possible confounding factors.

The most appropriate form of multivariate analysis for the purposes of this particular study was 'Discriminant Analysis'. Discriminant analysis takes simultaneous account of a large number of potentially-determining 'independent' variables in predicting a nominated 'dependent' variable, and it shows which of the independent variables remain significantly predictive when all the others have been taken into account. This method has a special virtue in that it can handle both 'categorical' (e.g. marital status) and 'quantitative' (e.g. maternal age) independent variables in a single analysis. Its primary function is to predict one 'dependent' variable – a categorical variable nominated by the investigator – in terms of loadings (i.e. coefficients) applied to all of the others The dependent variables to be predicted here were the health problems

TABLE 5.1

Variables included in discriminant analysis

Variable	Method of inclusion (0/1 . . . etc)
Parity	Primiparous/multiparous
Maternal age at booking	Continuous (years)
Marital status	Not married/married
Social class	I, II/III, IV, V
Ethnic group	Non Asian/Asian
Maternal height (ex = 748)	Continuous (centimetres)
Maternal hypertension (HBP)	No HBP/HBP
Ante-partum haemorrhage (APH)	No APH/APH
Induction of labour	Non-induced/induced
Multiple pregnancy	Singleton/multiple
Duration 1st stage of labour (ex = 273)	Continuous: (minutes)
Duration 2nd stage of labour (ex = 84)	Continuous: (minutes)
Type of fetal presentation	Atypical/occipito anterior
Forceps delivery	No forceps/forceps
Caesarean section	No section/section
Episiotomy	No episiotomy/episiotomy
Laceration	No laceration/laceration
Post-partum haemorrhage (PPH)	No PPH/PPH
Gestation at delivery	Term/pre-term
Epidural anaesthesia	No epidural/epidural
General anaesthesia (GA)	No GA/GA
Pethidine	No pethidine/pethidine
Inhalation analgesia	No inhalation/inhalation
Tranquillisers	No tranquillisers/tranquillisers
Spinal block	No spinal/spinal
Pudendal block	No pudendal/pudendal
Birthweight	Continuous (kilograms)
Head circumference (ex = 72)	Continuous (centimetres)
Length (ex = 200)	Continuous (centimetres)
Admission to special care (SCBU)	No SCBU/SCBU
Breast feeding on discharge	No breast feeding/breast feeding

*ex=n refers to numbers with missing data or inappropriate criteria

reported by the women on their questionnaires. Most of the variables used in the study, whether dependent or independent, were entered into the discriminant analysis as binary-categorical variables; for example . . . no epidural = 0, epidural = 1. A few, such as maternal age, duration of labour, birthweight of infant, although condensed into categories for ease of presentation in many of the tables, were recorded for discriminant analysis as continuous quantitative variables. The particular entry format for each of the variables is shown in Table 5.1.

The particular variant of discriminant analysis adopted for our purpose, selects variables in a stepwise manner, beginning with the one displaying the highest significance level (F-value); then the next highest . . . and so on. Only variables having an F-value of 3.84 or more, representing the 5% significance level, were listed. When all such primary predictors were identified and listed, the analysis was regarded as complete. Interpretation nevertheless calls for some caution.

Multi-way tabulations

The discriminant analysis for each health problem indicated which factors represented primary independent predictors. One of the hazards of statistical multivariate analysis relates to the possible presence of non-linear relationships, for example with maternal age or duration of labour. If the relationship with a particular symptom is non-linear, for example with an excess of symptoms at both ends of the range, this could obscure the results of the analysis. There can also be a problem with very closely related independent variables, such as Caesarean section and general anaesthesia, or forceps delivery and the duration of second stage labour. In addition there might be specific groups of the population, such as Asian women, where the relationships with symptoms differ greatly from those in the rest of the sample.

There were also practical reasons for testing whether the effects of individual predictors were widespread, or else localised to specific sub-groups or particular sets of circumstances. In order to do this and in view of the possible hazards of complete reliance on discriminate analysis, we completed complex sets of cross-tabulations of several of the symptom predictors. This particular form of analysis confirmed and refined the discriminant analyses, and moved us further towards the identification of the potential symptom determinants.

Technical data problems

Five items of information from the maternity case-notes were not recorded for all the women. All were quantitative items, namely maternal height, duration of first and second stages of labour, and the head circumference and length of the infant. The items were missing in 6.4%, 2.3%, 0.7%, 0.6% and 1.7% of cases respectively. We handled these omissions as seemed fit for each particular item. For maternal height and infant's head circumference and length, where a normal distribution curve would be expected, the missing values were replaced by the mean value for the sample and the amended records entered into the discriminant analyses. For the durations of the stages of labour, the form of the distribution in the total sample was such that this procedure was probably not legitimate and we thought it better simply to omit the whole record from any analyses which used these variables, rather than risk introducing bias. This meant that in some of the analyses the total number of women included was less than the full 11,701.

We encountered a special problem relating to 'Caesarean Section' and 'Duration of Labour'. Women who had a section did not have a genuine and comparable 'Duration of Labour'. Even for emergency sections which were preceded by a period of labour duration was not recorded. Under these rules, Caesarean section and duration of labour were mutually exclusive variables, never to be included within the same record, and could not be used within the same discriminant analysis. In these situations we carried out two separate discriminant analyses. The first was limited to vaginal deliveries and used duration of labour as a potential predictive variable. The other related to all births, including both Caesarean and vaginal deliveries; it used Caesarean section as a qualitative predictive variable, but excluded duration of labour. In practice the two forms of analysis often supplied useful complementary information on the genesis of particular health problems, and we shall report on these results in later chapters as we encounter them.

For most of the discriminant analyses carried out in the course of this investigation, the dependent variables were those individual health problems which met defined criteria of onset and duration. (These inclusion criteria are described in detail in Chapter 7). In general these were health problems occurring for the first time in the womans life within three months of the nominated delivery, and lasting for more than six weeks. The first stipulation was included in order to maximise the specificity of association between the symptoms and the events of the 'index' delivery. Unfortunately, the systematic exclusion of 'non-first-time' symptoms created an artificially biased association between symptom-occurrences and primiparity. A multiparous woman has more chance of having had a childbirth-related symptom before; her exclusion from the 'affected' group then creates a false relative symptom excess among primiparae. Sometimes, this carried over to produce a parallel bias in relation to maternal age, since older women too would have had more chance of experiencing symptoms – including non-childbirth related symptoms – on a previous occasion. In order to clarify these possibly spurious associations we have, where necessary, conducted additional discriminant analyses to predict the occurrence of symptoms **irrespective** of whether they had also been experienced on a previous occasion. That is, the analysis was repeated using **all** symptoms experienced within three months of the delivery and lasting more than six weeks, including both recurrent and continuous symptoms as well as the new occurrences. However, these investigations were carried out in a strictly supplementary sense, apart from the mainstream of analysis, and we shall comment upon them as we come to them.

Chapter 6 – Maternal, Obstetric and Anaesthetic Factors, and their Relationships

In this chapter we describe the circumstances and events preceding and surrounding childbirth, preparing the ground for identifying the potential origins of long-term health problems. We describe the social and demographic characteristics of the women enrolled into the study and the manner in which they varied. We describe the circumstances of the deliveries, and the obstetric and anaesthetic procedures employed. And we examine the relationships between them, identifying those which tended to occur together.

Where published data are available we consider the representativeness of our sample both against the general maternity population of Birmingham and against the population of England and Wales. Information relating to all Birmingham births up to 1984 was available from a research register held in the Department of Social Medicine at the University of Birmingham. Data on births in England and Wales were obtained from national Birth Statistics and from the Hospital In-patient Enquiry (H.I.P.E.) Maternity Statistics for 1977-81, and 1982-85, published by the Office of Population Censuses and Surveys (OPCS: 1986; 1988; 1989).

Social and demographic factors

The social and demographic make-up of the sample is detailed in Figure 6.1. This gives the distributions of the women within the sample according to parity, maternal age, marital status, social class, ethnic group and maternal height. The relationships between each of these socio-demographic factors are shown in detailed tabulations in Appendix 2, but the main outline and a number of illustrative relationships are described below.

Parity. Over a third of the women in our sample (35.8%) had delivered their first baby: 39.9% their second: 16.9% their third: 5.1% their fourth: and 2.3% a later child. Information on all Birmingham births over a similar period, showed that 39.9% of women had delivered a first baby; 30.5% a second; 15.2% a third; 7.1% a fourth and 7.2% a subsequent child. The main difference was that the study sample had a relative deficiency of first births, a greater proportion of second births and fewer fifth or subsequent births. Figures for England and Wales for parity are published only for married women. The proportion of first babies over the eight year period was also greater than in our sample, at 41% (OPCS 1989).

Figure 6.1

Socio-Demographic Variable-Distribution

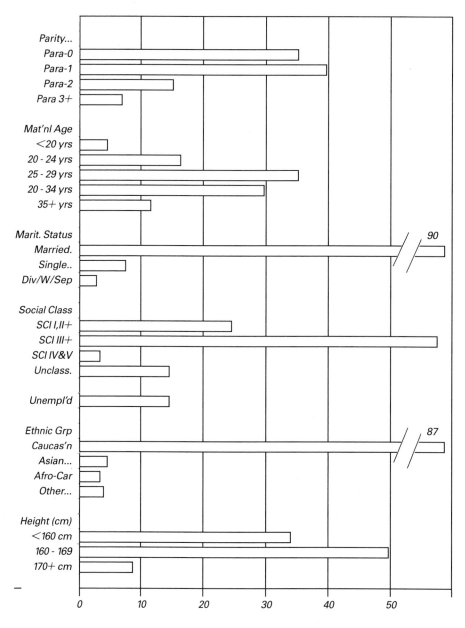

Percent in Class.

Maternal age. The ages of the women in the study sample at the time of hospital booking ranged from 12 to 52 years. Most, 55%, were between 20 and 29 years, with another 30% aged 30 to 34 years. Only 4.3% were under 20 years and 12% were aged 35 or more. The mean age was 28 years. The sample contained more older women and fewer under 20's than did either births in Birmingham or in the country as a whole. Birth statistics for England and Wales averaged over the eight year period, showed 65% of women delivering at age 20-29; 9% under 20 years; 19% at 30-34; and 7% aged 35 years or more. In Birmingham the comparisons were 63% delivering at age 20-29 years; 12% under 20; 18% aged 30-34 and 7%, 35 or more.

Maternal age was closely related to parity, first births being much more common among younger mothers: 37% of first births in the sample were to women under 25 years compared with only 14% of subsequent births.

Marital status. The majority of our respondents (89.9%) were married; 7.8% were single and the remaining 2.3% were separated, widowed or divorced. In England and Wales the proportion of births to unmarried women almost doubled over the eight year study period, from 10.2% in 1978 to 19.2% in 1985; the average between 1978 and 1985 was 14% compared with the 10.1% in our sample.

In the maternity case-notes, information relating to marital status was recorded at the hospital antenatal booking visit and a subsequent change in status was not routinely recorded. A number of women categorised as unmarried will have been married before the delivery; we have no data on this proportion in this sample, but in a previous (unrelated) study based on a population at the same hospital in 1981-82 (MacArthur et al 1985) it amounted to about 15% of those actually categorised as unmarried. The proportion unmarried, nationally and in the sample, probably differ even more than the above figures suggest.

Marital status was related both to age and to parity: 62% of unmarried women in the sample were under 25 years, and 60% had delivered their first baby.

Social class. The social class categories in our sample were based upon the Registrar General's classification of the occupation of the husband, as recorded in the maternity case-notes. Single women, and women whose husbands were unemployed or were students, were not classified. Among the 15.1% unclassified cases the woman was single in 7%*, the occupation of the husband not known in 2.9%, the husband unemployed in 4.5%, and a student in 0.7%. A

---

*Occasionally in the case of young, single girls still living with parents, their father's occupation was used to place them in a social class. This accounts for the smaller proportion recorded as single here compared with the recording for marital status.

high proportion of the sample (11.4%) were social class I, with 13.3% in social class II. The largest group was social class III, with 57.3% This group had not been subdivided into manual and non-manual sub-categories. Only 2.9% of the women were categorised as social class IV or V. This distribution is quite different to Birmingham as a whole, where only 3% of women were categorised as social class I, much less than in our sample, and another 11% as social class II. Birmingham births had far more social class IV (17%) and V (5%) women, with 47% in social class III.

National proportions according to the social class of the father as published, are based only on births within marriage. Over the eight year period, 29% were social class I and II, which was comparable with our own re-calculated within-marriage proportion of 27%. The main differences related to social classes III, IV and V: 21% were in classes IV and V compared with our 3%, with 47% in social class III compared with our own 62%.

Social class was closely associated with maternal age: only 5% of the social class I and II women in the sample were under 25 years compared with 21% of social classes III, IV and V.

Ethnic group. Ethnic group was defined in the maternity case-notes according to the mother's 'ethnic origin' rather than 'country of birth'. Ethnic origin was as perceived by hospital registration staff, based upon name, colour and dress, as well as statements made by the mother herself. The majority of the births (87%) were to Caucasian mothers, almost all (84% of all births) being British. A further 5% were Asian, most of whom were categorised as Indian or Pakistani, with only thirty-eight women categorised as 'other Asian'. Another 3.5% were Afro-Caribbean and 4.5% were of 'other races'. In England and Wales the statistics over the eight year period averaged 91% of births to Caucasian, 4.5% to Asian and 2.5% to Afro-Caribbean women. In national statistics, however, ethnic group is defined according to mother's country of birth. In Birmingham as a whole the definition was the same as in our sample but the ethnic mix was completely different, with only 66% of births to Caucasian mothers during the years 1978-85, whilst 24% were to Asian and 7% to Afro-Caribbean women.

Ethnic comparisons with the other socio-demographic factors in our own sample also showed that the Asian women contained in it were atypical of the city as a whole. In Birmingham as a whole fewer of the Asian mothers were primiparous and from the higher social classes than the Caucasians. In our sample however equal proportions of Asian and Caucasian women had delivered their first baby and the proportion of Asian women in social classes I and II was not substantially lower.

On the other hand the few Afro-Caribbean women in our sample, differed from the Caucasian women in almost all social and demographic respects.

Differences in age and marital status were particularly striking; as many as 51% of the Afro-Caribbean compared with 21% of Caucasian mothers were less than 25 years of age and only 42% were married.

Symptom differences however for the Afro-Caribbean women were in general much smaller than for the Asian women. Because of this and also because of the small numbers in this group, we have made little further reference to Afro-Caribbean women.

Maternal height. In our sample, 34% of the women were under 160 cms in height; 50% were between 160 and 169 cms in height and 9% were 170 cms or more. Maternal height was not recorded for 7%. No national or other local figures are available for comparison.

Height was closely related to social class: 33% of the tallest women (170 cms or more) were in social classes I or II but only 20% of the shortest women (under 160 cms).

Obstetric and anaesthetic factors

The circumstances of the delivery and the use of obstetric procedures are shown in Figure 6.2, while details of anaesthetic and pain relief procedures are given in Figure 6.3. Detailed tabulations of the cross-relationships between all these factors and between the socio-demographic characteristics described earlier are given in Appendix 2. Some examples of these relationships and comparisons where available with national and local figures, are described below.

Hypertension. A total of 1055 women (9%) in the sample had a record in their case notes of hypertension and/or proteinuria. Eighty-six of these were labelled as having chronic or essential hypertension, nineteen of whom had gestational hypertension and/or proteinuria superimposed. Gestational hypertension alone was recorded in a further 714 and another 140 had recorded proteinuria as well. Severe pre-eclampsia, sufficient to result in admission to intensive care, was recorded in 42 women. There were also 73 women recorded as having proteinuria but with no hypertension. National figures for hypertension are reported without subdivisions: in 1980, 9.8% were categoriesed as having hypertension and in 1985 the proportion was 8.8% This is similar to our own proportion of 9%.

Hypertension was more frequent in primiparous (12%) than in multiparous women (7%); Asian and Afro-Caribbean women had lower rates (5% and 4% respectively) than Caucasians (9%).

Ante-partum haemorrhage (APH) was recorded in 327 women in the study population (2.8%). They included 47 (0.4%) with placenta praevia, 67 (0.6%) with abruptio placentae and 213 (1.8%) with some other form of ante-partum

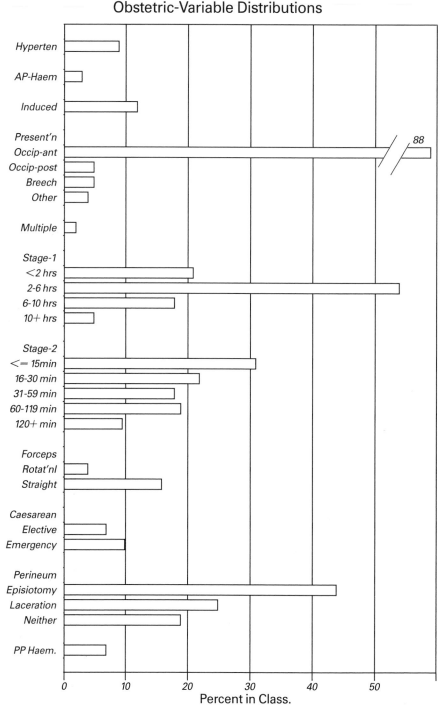

Figure 6.2
Obstetric-Variable Distributions

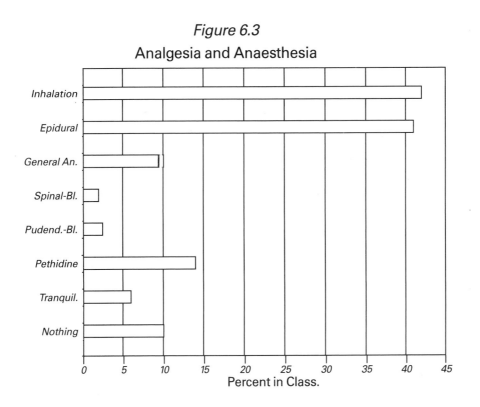

Figure 6.3

Analgesia and Anaesthesia

haemorrhage. The proportions with APH in the country as a whole were similar, 3.1% in both 1980 and 1985.

Ante-partum haemorrhage was more frequent in older women: 3.7% among those aged 30 or more. Many APH's (41%) resulted in delivery by Caesarean section (see later).

Onset of labour. Labour was induced in 1434 women (12.3%) and another 975 (8.3%) were coded as having an elective Caesarean section, prior to the onset of labour. Of these 975, 770 were true 'elective' sections while the others were emergency sections carried out for a problem arising suddenly sometime before labour began (See Chapter 4). The remainder of the women were delivered following either a spontaneous onset or a spontaneous/augmented onset. Prostaglandin pessaries were not reported in the case-notes as inductions. National figures for inductions were 20.2% in 1980 and 17.5% in 1985: higher than in our group.

Women with hypertension were much more likely to have an induction: 39% compared with 9% in those with no hypertension. The most frequent form of pain relief in induced labour was epidural anaesthesia, used in 66% of induced compared with 36% of spontaneous labours.

Fetal presentation. The majority of fetal presentations in the sample were occipito-anterior (87.7%), with 4.4% occipito-posterior, 4.4% breech, and 1.9% lateral; other atypical presentations accounted for the remaining 1.5%.

Atypical fetal presentation was associated with primiparity, occurring in 15% of first births compared with 10.6% of subsequent births. Again, epidural anaesthesia was a common form of pain relief with atypical fetal presentations and was used in 59% of such cases.

Multiple deliveries. There were 169 women who had multiple deliveries (1.4%): 163 sets of twins and 6 sets of triplets. This proportion is greater than either the national or the Birmingham figures, both 1.0%. This may result from the higher proportion of older women in our sample; also the fact that the hospital has the Regional Specialty Neonatal Unit.

Multiple pregnancies were more likely to have hypertension during pregnancy (19%) and to have induced labours (21%); 66% had epidural anaesthesia.

Stages of labour. The separate stages of labour were recorded in the maternity case-notes in hours and minutes and entered to the computer file in this continuous format. They are condensed for presentation purposes into duration-bands, as shown in Table 6.1. The first stage of labour begins with the onset of regular painful contractions, maternally defined, and is complete when the cervix is fully dilated. It is sometimes referred to as the 'active' stage in order to separate it from the earlier more 'latent' phase. The second stage begins at full dilatation and is completed at the delivery of the child. The time of onset of labour is generally declared by the woman, while the transition to second stage is determined by clinical staff. Durations of first stages were recorded for all but 273 (2.3%), and second stages for all but 84 (0.7%), of vaginal deliveries. For women having a Caesarean section, there was no coding of duration of labour, even when the section was an emergency procedure carried out in mid-labour.

Among the vaginal deliveries 5.4% of first stages lasted less than one hour, 15.6% one to two hours, 53.8% between two and under six hours, 17.2% from six to under ten hours and 5.2% ten hours or longer. Among second stages, 30.8% lasted fifteen minutes or less, 21.9% between sixteen and thirty minutes, 17.9% between thirty-one and fifty-nine minutes, 18.9% between one and under two hours, and 9.6% for two hours or longer.

There was a close correlation between the duration of the first and second stages, with 91% of the short first stages (under two hours) being followed by short second stages (under one hour); compared with only 49% where first stage lasted six hours or more. Primiparous women had much longer first and second

TABLE 6.1

Duration of first and second stages of labour

Duration of first stage	No.	% of all deliveries	% of vaginal deliveries
Under 1 hour	529	(4.5)	(5.4)
1 – 1 hr 59 mins	1525	(13.0)	(15.6)
2 – 3 hrs 59 mins	3215	(27.5)	(32.9)
4 – 5 hrs 59 mins	2049	(17.5)	(20.9)
6 – 7 hrs 59 mins	1138	(9.7)	(11.6)
8 – 9 hrs 59 mins	546	(4.7)	(5.6)
10 hours or more	511	(4.4)	(5.2)
Not known	273	(2.3)	(2.8)
Total vaginal deliveries	9785		(100)
Sections	1915	(16.4)	
Total	11701	(100)	

Duration of second stage	No.	% of all deliveries	% of vaginal deliveries
Up to 5 mins	593	(5.1)	(6.1)
6 – 10 mins	1284	(11.0)	(13.1)
11 – 15 mins	1137	(9.7)	(11.6)
16 – 30 mins	2142	(18.3)	(21.9)
31 – 59 mins	1748	(14.9)	(17.9)
1 hr – 1 hr 30 mins	1139	(9.7)	(11.6)
1 hr 31 mins – 1 hr 59 mins	719	(6.1)	(7.3)
2 hrs – 2 hrs 59 mins	737	(6.3)	(7.5)
3 hours or more	203	(1.7)	(2.1)
Not known	84	(0.7)	(0.8)
Total vaginal deliveries	9785		(100)
Sections	1915	(16.4)	
Total	11701	(100)	

stage labours: they were three times as likely as multiparae to have a first stage of six hours or more, and four times as likely to have a second stage of one hour or more.

Obstetric procedures. Forceps were employed in 19.7% of all deliveries in the sample. Most (15.9%) were straight (non-rotational) forceps, but 3.8% were rotational. There were a further 146 breech deliveries with forceps applied to the after-coming head, and 42 ventouse deliveries, but these are excluded from the general forceps category. This is a much higher rate of forceps than for the country overall. The national forceps rates ranged from 13.1% in 1978 to 9.1% in 1985 with an eight year mean of 10.7%. It is also higher than among Birmingham births during the relevant period, where 13% were categorised under 'all instrumental deliveries'.

Forceps were used more frequently for the delivery of a first baby: 36% compared with 10% of later babies. Afro-Caribbean women had lower rates (9%) than Caucasians (20%), even though more of them had delivered first babies. Use of forceps was closely associated with long labour, occurring in 56% of deliveries where second stage was one hour or more.

Caesarean section was employed in 16.4% of the sample deliveries, comprising 9.8% emergency sections and 6.6% elective sections. As with forceps, the Caesarean section rate was much greater than rates in the country as a whole, which ranged from 7.5% in 1978 to 10.5% in 1985, with a mean of 9.4%. The Caesarean section rate for all Birmingham births was similar to the national rate, at 9.9%. Taking forceps and sections together, 36.1% of the women in the study sample had one or the other: the national proportion was only 20.1%.

Caesarean sections, especially electives, were more than twice as frequent among shorter mothers; in 21% of women under 160 cms compared with 9% of women of 170 cms or more. Ante-natal complications also resulted in higher section rates: 30% where hypertension was present and 41% following antepartum haemorrhage.

Episiotomies were performed on 5112 women (43.7%) and lacerations were recorded in 2907 (24.8%). A few of these women (67) had both episiotomy and laceration. The episiotomy rate in the sample was much greater after a forceps delivery, at 96%. Third degree tears (i.e. involving perineal muscle) were recorded in twenty-nine women. Only 32% of the whole sample (3749) had an intact perineum after delivery and many of them because they had a Caesarean section: only 18.7% of women who delivered vaginally had neither an episiotomy nor laceration. National figures are reported only for episiotomies, not lacerations: in 1980, 52% of women had an episiotomy; in 1985 this proportion had fallen to 36.6%.

Post-partum haemorrhage (PPH). A total of 1487 women (12.7%) in our sample were recorded as having a primary post-partum haemorrhage – defined as an estimated blood loss of more than 500ml. Sixty-two (0.5%) women had a secondary post-partum haemorrhage, 15 of whom also had a primary one. Our main analyses (later) refer only to primary PPH.

The 500ml criteria was properly applied, in fact, only to vaginal deliveries. After a section the 'normal' blood loss has been estimated as 750 to 1000ml; yet only 41.5% of sections also had a coded PPH. The coding is probably meaningful only for vaginal deliveries, where 7.1% had a record of PPH.

The national figures for post-partum haemorrhage were only 2% in 1980 and 2.1% in 1985. The difference may be due in part to different rates of Caesarean section, and to variations in individual interpretation.

Analgesia and anaesthesia. The most commonly recorded form of pain relief was inhalation analgesia,* in 42% of the women; this was followed closely by epidural anaesthesia in 40.7%. A general anaesthetic was given to 9.9%, 1.4% had a spinal block and 2.4% a pudendal block. Pethidine was given to 14.2% of the women and tranquillisers were recorded in 5.8%. Many women had more than one form of analgesia or anaesthesia; but 10% had nothing at all recorded.

Data are collected nationally as part of the H.I.P.E. maternity statistics on the types of analgesia and anaesthesia used during delivery, but they are not published. This is said to be because the figures are not considered reliable. For epidural anaesthesia, in particular, usage will certainly vary according to the level of 'anaesthetic cover' available within different maternity units. A study of the availability of epidural anaesthesia by Hibbard and Scott (1990), using annual statistical returns to the Hospital Recognition Committee, showed a mean usage rate over 271 units between 1982-86 of 17%. Regional rates ranged from 10.1% in N.E. Thames to 26% in Trent: the average for the West Midlands was 14.9%. Only 3.7% of the units had a rate of more than 40%.

These different forms of analgesia and anaesthesia were inter-related with each other and with other factors. Epidurals were used more often for first births (56%) than for subsequent ones (32%): and in induced labours (66%), in multiple pregnancies (66%) and in forceps deliveries (79%). Inhalation analgesia was used more in 'normal' deliveries. Pudendal block was four times as likely to be given in atypical than in occipito-anterior fetal presentations; 80% of pudendal blocks were given for forceps deliveries. Spinal block, although infrequently given, was eight times as likely where the second stage lasted for an hour or more, compared with durations of up to fifteen minutes. All but forty-three of the 1158 general anaesthetics were given for Caesarean sections.

*This refers to pre-mixed 50/50 nitrous oxide and oxygen.

Women who had no analgesia or anaesthesia were more likely to have had short labours, especially second stages: with a second stage of fifteen minutes or less, 21.4% had no pain relief compared with only 2.4% where it lasted an hour or more.

The infant. Recorded gestations at delivery ranged from 24 weeks up to 45 weeks. Of the 800 women (6.8%) in the sample who had a pre-term delivery (before 37 weeks), 25 had delivered before 28 weeks: 245 between 28 and 34 weeks: and the remaining 530 between 34 and 37 weeks. Pre-term infants were much more likely to have been delivered by Caesarean section: 39% compared with 15% of full term deliveries.

The mean birthweight of the infants in this sample was 3334 grams. There were 6.6% who weighed 2500 grams or less; 30.9% between 2501 and 3000 grams, 32.1% between 3001 and 3600 grams and 30.4% were heavier. Mean head circumference was 34 cms: 11.3% measured 32 cms or less, most (67%) were 33 to 35 cms and 21% were over 35 cms. Head circumference was not recorded for 72 infants. The mean length of the babies was 51 cms: 11.4% were up to 47 cms in length, 54.3% between 47 and 52 cms, and 32.6% were more than 52cms. Length was not recorded for 200 infants. (1.7%).

Birthweight, length and head circumference were all related to parity: for example 44% of babies weighing up to 2500 grams were first births compared with 29% of those over 3600 grams. Asian and Afro-Caribbean women were less likely to delivery heavier babies: only 12.8% of Asian and 17.8% of Afro-Caribbean mothers delivered babies weighing over 3600 grams, compared with 31.8% of Caucasians. Among babies of 2500 grams or less, 63% were pre-term. Low birthweight was also associated with ante-partum haemorrhage, which occurred in 9.9% of those weighing 2500 grams or less compared with 1.5% of those weighing over 3600 grams. Head circumference and length were closely correlated with weight.

One in ten of the infants (1256, 9.9%) delivered in the sample were admitted to the Special Care Baby Unit (SCBU), with babies weighing 2500 grams or less comprising 52% of all admissions. Length of stay ranged from one day (233) up to twenty-four weeks. Almost half (46.3%) were discharged within one week but 173 (13.8%) stayed for more than four weeks.

Breast feeding at the time of discharge from hospital was recorded in 7937 infants (67.8%), of whom 238 also received artificial supplements. Breast feeding was more frequent among social class I and II women (84%) than in the other social classes (64%).

Perinatal deaths were excluded from the sample in order to avoid distress to mothers. This will have resulted in a disproportionate reduction in early gestations, low birthweights and SCBU admissions.

Inter-correlations

Many of the factors described in the previous paragraphs were strongly inter-correlated with each other. We have given examples throughout, but there were many others. It was not possible to devise a form of presentation showing all these inter-correlations which would be both concise and intelligible. A simple correlation table would be at the very least unwieldy. We have therefore used the device of presenting a separate tabulation for each factor, in which associations are given with every other factor. However, since the chief use of this will be for reference purposes at a later stage of the analysis, we have relegated this to an appendix (Appendix 2).

We give below two detailed examples of inter-relationships in order to illustrate the complexities of the data, and the care that is required in moving from the simple detection of statistical associations between pairs of factors to inferring the potential determinants of later health problems.

Example 1

Parity comparisons given in Table A2.1 show that virtually all the social, obstetric and anaesthetic factors vary according to whether the birth is a first or a subsequent one. This has wide implications for other inter-relationships. For example, first births more frequently had long labours: 55% of primiparous women had a second stage lasting one hour or more, compared with only 14% of multiparous women. Table A2.18 compares deliveries with and without epidural anaesthesia and the first association shown is with parity: 49% of epidural deliveries were first births compared with only 27% of non-epidural deliveries. Not surprisingly therefore, women with epidurals have longer labours. 54% of epidural labours had a second stage of an hour or more, compared with only 12% of labours without an epidural. How do we interpret this? Does epidural anaesthesia prolong labour: or do long labours invoke epidurals: or is there merely an indirect statistical association via the parity relationship, without any casual implication? If relationships are subsequently found between particular health problems and any of these factors, the same problems of interpretation will recur. We will always have to ask which associations are primary and which are indirect and secondary.

Example 2

Perineal complications are shown on Table A2.16. There are three main categories; episiotomy (where the perineum is cut); laceration (where the perineum tears) and an intact perineum. The most direct of the associations is between an intact perineum and Caesarean section, and this association will produce various indirect statistical associations: thus, an intact perineum is found more frequently following pre-term deliveries, low infant birthweight and with special care admission. Episiotomy is frequently used in forceps deliveries and 43% of all episiotomies occurred in these circumstances. This results in secondary associations between episiotomy and primiparity (since more primiparae have forceps); and between episiotomy and longer labours (since forceps are used more commonly after longer labours). Many of the statistical associations of episiotomy are also clearly indirect. This again exemplifies the hazards of inferring true relationships with post partum health problems, without first undertaking detailed additional multivariate analyses.

Discussion

This chapter describes the study sample in terms of the social, demographic, obstetric and anaesthetic characteristics of the women included. For some factors, comparisons were possible with all Birmingham births and with births in the country at large (usually England and Wales). The sample differed from both local and national populations with respect to maternal age and social class, with an excess of older women and class I and II women. The ethnic mix differed little from the national picture but there were considerable local differences. In particular there were far fewer Asian mothers in the sample than in Birmingham births overall, and these Asian mothers in the sample were socially atypical of Asian women in Birmingham as a whole. Among the obstetric procedures, forceps and sections were more frequent in our sample than nationally or locally, but the episiotomy rate was similar and the induction rate was lower. The proportions with hypertension and ante-partum haemorrhage were comparable, but our sample recorded greater numbers with post-partum haemorrhage.

This investigation has two main purposes, and the contrasts with national data are relevant to one of them, but not the other. The first purpose is to describe the nature and the frequencies of long-term health problems following childbirth; the second is to seek out their potential determinants. The differences between our sample and the general population have little or no significance for the second of these purposes, but demand modification of our estimates of the frequencies of symptoms, when extrapolating to the country as a whole. The differences affect all numeral appraisals of the relative importance of particular health problems in the country as a whole. For example, if we show that higher maternal age is a predictor of a symptom, (say stress incontinence), then because our population contained more older women, the proportion of post-partum stress incontinence which could be attributed to this factor in the country as a whole would be less than in our sample. Conversely, if vaginal delivery was found to be an important predictor of stress incontinence, then the post-partum prevalence of this condition would be greater in England and Wales than would appear from our study, where proportionally more Caesarean sections were carried out.

These effects will be discussed in a later chapter. Here we simply set out the nature of the overall problem. Our next tasks, in the chapters following are to describe the overall pattern of morbidity and then to describe the frequencies and examine the predictors of each of the different health problems about which we enquired.

Chapter 7 – The Nature, Frequencies and Durations of Health Problems

In this chapter we describe the overall results of the questionnaire-based enquiry. It complements the descriptions of the maternity case-note data of the previous chapter. We set out the information provided by the women about their health, and the frequencies of different symptoms occurring after the index delivery – the most recent delivery at the maternity hospital from which the sample was drawn. The intervals since the nominated deliveries ranged from thirteen months to nine years. The women were asked to note their subsequent experience of each of a list of 25 different symptoms or health problems listed on the questionnaire form, and then to answer an 'open' question. The list of health problems as shown on the questionnaire is in Appendix 1 and in Table 7.1.

Some of the listed symptoms, such as postnatal depression or stress incontinence, were suspected on prior grounds of being associated with childbirth, or even with specific obstetric procedures. Some, such as dental problems, bowel upsets and indigestion were included mainly for 'control' purposes and as 'negative checks' with regard to general over-reporting after particular types of deliveries or as a result of neurotic or hyperchondriacal tendencies. In general we made sure that all parts of the body, as well as varying categories of symptoms were represented.

For each symptom or health problem on the questionnaire the women were asked first whether they had experienced the problem since having the index baby. If they had, they were then asked: had they ever had it before the birth? how long after the birth, had the symptom first occurred? When had it stopped? and had they sought medical advice and received any treatment? (Questionnaire shown in Appendix 1).

Frequencies of health problems

Overall frequencies

Table 7.1 gives the numbers and proportions (Column 1) of women who said they had experienced each of the various health problems at any time since the nominated delivery. Figure 7.1 also shows this in diagrammatic form. Altogether, 9722 women (83.1%) reported one or more of the listed symptoms. Certain classes of problem affected very substantial proportions of the women. They included backache, urinary stress incontinence and frequency,

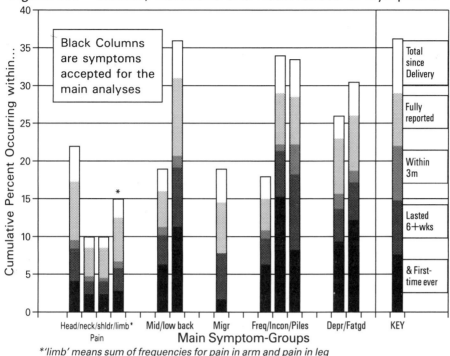

Figure 7.1 Onsets, Durations and Recurrences of Symptoms

Cumulative Percent Occurring within...

Black Columns are symptoms accepted for the main analyses

KEY:
Total since Delivery
Fully reported
Within 3m
Lasted 6+wks
& First-time ever

Main Symptom-Groups

Head/neck/shldr/limb* Pain   Mid/low back   Migr   Freq/Incon/Piles   Depr/Fatgd   KEY

*'limb' means sum of frequencies for pain in arm and pain in leg

haemorrhoids, depression and anxiety, extreme tiredness, and frequent headaches and migraine.

The true proportions of women suffering the different post-partum symptoms within this time limit were certainly greater than these figures show, because some women were unable to specify the exact times of onset (see Column 5 of Table 7.1), and these symptoms were excluded.

Occurrence within three post-partum months

Because the study covered a long period since delivery, up to nine years in some cases, many women would have experienced certain of these symptoms at times unrelated to their deliveries. We therefore restricted our more detailed analyses to those symptoms which had started 'within three months' of the delivery.

Even with this constraint, 70.5% of the women recorded at least one symptom. The detailed results are shown in the second column of Table 7.1, and in Figure 7.1. It was clear that some symptoms (e.g. backache, stress incontinence, piles) were more specifically associated with onsets in the first three months than were others (e.g. pain in arms, tingling in hands or feet, buzzing in ears,

TABLE 7.1

Frequency of health problems reported after 11,701 deliveries

	1 Total occurring since delivery	2 Total occurring within 3 months of delivery	3 Occurring within 3 mths of delivery: duration over 6 wks.	4 Occurring within 3 mths of delivery: never had it before: duration over 6 wks.	5 Occurred post delivery but don't know when started, ended or had before
	No. (%)	No. (%)	No. (%)	No. (%)	No. (%)
Frequent headaches	1967 (16.8)	1079 (9.2)	972 (8.3)	419 (3.6)	545 (4.7)
Neckache	979 (8.4)	460 (3.9)	410 (3.5)	228 (1.9)	204 (1.7)
Shoulder ache	999 (8.5)	507 (4.3)	469 (4.0)	263 (2.2)	204 (1.7)
Ache in middle of back	1942 (16.6)	1306 (11.2)	1184 (10.1)	719 (6.1)	336 (2.9)
Ache in bottom of back	3602 (30.8)	2382 (20.4)	2191 (18.7)	1266 (10.8)	576 (4.9)
Pain in arms	456 (3.9)	199 (1.7)	186 (1.6)	108 (0.9)	88 (0.8)
Pain in legs	1037 (8.9)	603 (5.2)	506 (4.3)	240 (2.1)	187 (1.6)
Weakness in arms	460 (3.9)	232 (2.0)	210 (1.8)	142 (1.2)	107 (0.9)
Weakness in legs	502 (4.3)	320 (2.7)	247 (2.1)	148 (1.3)	77 (0.7)
Bowel upsets	1128 (9.6)	714 (6.1)	550 (4.7)	321 (2.7)	212 (1.8)
Tingling in hands/fingers	1266 (10.8)	600 (5.1)	531 (4.5)	293 (2.5)	290 (2.5)
Tingling in feet/toes	472 (4.0)	260 (2.2)	223 (1.9)	126 (1.1)	81 (0.7)
Buzzing in ears	467 (4.0)	192 (1.6)	170 (1.5)	76 (0.6)	156 (1.3)
Flashing lights/spots	987 (8.4)	525 (4.5)	467 (4.0)	174 (1.5)	248 (2.1)
Dizziness/fainting	932 (8.0)	486 (4.2)	406 (3.5)	211 (1.8)	215 (1.8)
Migraine	1756 (15.0)	857 (7.3)	827 (7.1)	165 (1.4)	466 (4.0)
Indigestion	858 (7.3)	440 (3.8)	409 (3.5)	127 (1.1)	229 (2.0)

TABLE 7.1 – *continued*

Urinary frequency	1760 (15.0)	1198 (9.4)	1104 (9.4)	668 (5.7)	390 (3.3)
Stress incontinence	3355 (28.7)	2507 (21.4)	2408 (20.6)	1782 (15.2)	619 (5.3)
High blood pressure	440 (3.8)	284 (2.4)	208 (1.8)	48 (0.4)	91 (0.8)
Haemorrhoids	3352 (28.6)	2540 (21.7)	2061 (17.6)	931 (8.0)	584 (5.0)
Varicose veins	1357 (11.6)	887 (7.6)	860 (7.3)	151 (1.3)	367 (3.1)
Dental problems	858 (7.3)	355 (3.0)	316 (2.7)	124 (1.1)	271 (2.3)
Depression/anxiety	2636 (22.5)	1790 (15.3)	1563 (13.4)	1065 (9.1)	360 (3.1)
Extreme tiredness	3027 (25.9)	2163 (18.5)	1999 (17.1)	1427 (12.2)	522 (4.5)
Other	937 (8.0)	633 (5.4)	555 (4.7)	423 (3.6)	77 (0.7)
No. of women with one or more of the above symptoms	9722 (83.1)	8250 (70.5)	7480 (63.9)	5457 (46.6)	
Total number of symptoms	37532	20695	21032	11645	7502

41

migraine). For most symptoms, the majority in fact started immediately after the delivery (see later).

Duration over six weeks

All women have contact with either their obstetrician or their general practitioner approximately six weeks after delivery, when they have their postnatal check, but there are no routine arrangements for longer-term follow-ups. This six week check is a practice of very long standing, and it is no doubt for this reason that systematic routine information on longer-lasting post-partum health problems is scarce. For many of the disorders which we recorded, the scientific literature is almost empty. It was mainly for this reason that we ourselves were especially concerned with the period beyond the postnatal check, with disorders extending beyond this time. In addition that many women might not recall symptoms of shorter duration after an interval of several years. For the purposes of our main investigations we therefore accepted only those symptoms which had lasted for more than six weeks. Column 3 of Table 7.1 shows the numbers of women meeting both of these acceptance criteria: that is who reported symptoms occurring within three months of delivery and lasting more than six weeks: a total of 63.9% reported at least one symptom so defined. It became evident on detailed examination of the responses that most of the symptoms had in fact persisted for much longer than six weeks (see later).

First time symptoms

One of the main objectives of the study was to identify relationships between the reported health problems and the recorded circumstances of a particular delivery. We therefore asked whether the symptoms had occurred for the first time following the nominated birth. We wished to separate long-standing health problems, those which had followed previous deliveries, and those that had started during the pregnancy, from those associated with the delivery for which we had detailed information. Column 4 of Table 7.1 gives the numbers, from among those in the previous column, which were 'first time' problems.

We realised that exclusion from the main analyses of symptoms that had occurred before, would have its costs. Some of the excluded symptoms might indeed have been relevant to aspects of the delivery. For example, a woman may have suffered backache in the past, perhaps following an injury, and then developed a different form of backache as a result of her delivery; yet this would be excluded. Stress incontinence may have occurred after a previous delivery and partly resolved, but recurred with greater severity following this delivery. This too would be excluded. The last example highlights a secondary problem;

the exclusion of all but newly occurring symptoms will necessarily result in the selective over-exclusion of any progressive forms of delivery-related ill-health among multiparous women. Since women of higher parities have had a greater chance of experiencing childbirth-related symptoms before, this selective exclusion could result in spurious statistical associations between these symptoms and primiparity. Older women will also have experienced some of the symptoms irrespective of childbirth, simply through the passage of time, and their selective exclusion might create a spurious excess in younger women. We shall consider these difficulties later.

Inadequately dated symptoms

Many women reported the occurrence of a health problem since delivering their child, but did not say when it started, or ended, or whether they had had it before: their numbers are in the final column of Table 7.1. We excluded these inadequately dated reports from our main analyses in order to maximise the specificity of the relationships between the symptoms and the circumstances and events of a particular birth. Some would anyway have only related to short-term symptoms and others might have started months or years after the delivery, but some should probably be counted within any assessment of the total morbidity of childbirth.

Relevant symptom group

Our main analyses are therefore restricted to accurately dated reports of conditions which had started within three months of the index delivery, persisted for more than six weeks, and had never been experienced by the woman before. These are listed in column 4 of Table 7.1 and shown in diagrammatic form in Figure 7.1 as the 'solid black' panel of the columns. Overall, 46.6% of the women in the sample (5475) reported at least one such symptom. The most frequently experienced complaints were middle (6.1%) and lower backache (10.8%), urinary stress incontinence (15.2%) and frequency (5.7%), depression and/or anxiety (9%), haemorrhoids (8%), extreme tiredness (12%) and frequent headaches (3.6%) or migraine (1.4%).

Figure 7.1 demonstrates clearly the small proportions (shown in black) of the totals, which were included in these analytical studies.

Although all these symptom frequencies relate to self-perceived problems, unconfirmed by further questioning or examination, this struck us as a truly remarkable level of morbidity, far beyond that which we had expected. It is even more remarkable, judging from the contrast between these observations and a sparse scientific literature, that no one seems to have noticed that so vast a problem exists, or even thought to ask. The formidable logistic problems of carrying out such a survey, described in Chapter 1, may provide part of the explanation.

Durations of health problems

The reported durations of the conditions are set out in detail in Table 7.2 and in diagrammatic form in Fig 7.2. We demanded a duration of more than six weeks for inclusion in our 'relevant symptom' group (Column 1). In fact the great majority, around 90%, had lasted more than three months (Column 2), and about 70% had lasted more than a year (Column 3). Many women, 60-70%, were still complaining of their symptoms at the time of our enquiry (Column 4, Table 7.2.), after an interval of thirteen months to nine years. These durations, we recall, do not include recurrence, continuation or exacerbation of symptoms already experienced before the birth.

The main exceptions to these very high rates of persistence were for depression/anxiety and extreme tiredness, where 'only' 27% and 39% of symptoms respectively were still present at the time of the enquiry. The majority of the other symptoms seem very often to have become truly chronic, such that the accumulated prevalence of post-partum morbidity within the population at large, must be enormous.

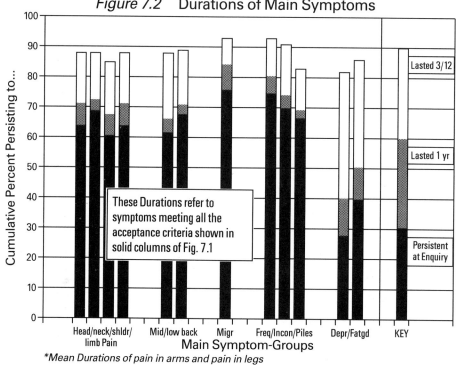

Figure 7.2   Durations of Main Symptoms

Mean Durations of pain in arms and pain in legs

Onsets of health problems

We included in the main analysis all new symptoms of over six weeks duration that started at any time within three months of the delivery. We supply evidence in later chapters to support the general appropriateness of this three month acceptance-rule, although the optimal limit varies a little for different symptoms. For most health problems the majority of onsets were within the first post-partum week. Figure 7.3 demonstrates this clearly. The numbers of first week onsets are also shown in Column 1 of Table 7.3; and Column 2 shows the numbers starting within four weeks. Column 3 gives the full total of those starting within the first three post-partum months, ie those included as the main analysis group.

Column 4 of Table 7.3 supplied some indication of the childbirth-specificity of particular symptoms, showing the proportions of new long-term symptoms which started at different times within the whole of the first year. If there was no relationship with childbirth we would expect roughly equal proportions of symptoms to start in each week throughout the year. Some symptoms followed very closely after the delivery; 81% of first-year stress incontinence, 79% of haemorrhoids and 76% of urinary frequency started within a week of the birth.

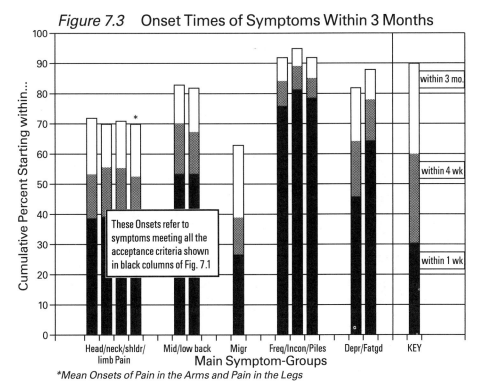

Figure 7.3 Onset Times of Symptoms Within 3 Months

*Mean Onsets of Pain in the Arms and Pain in the Legs

45

TABLE 7.2

Duration of health problems starting within three months of delivery and never experienced before

	1 Lasted over six weeks No. (%) of total sample	2 Lasted over 3 months No. (%) of 1	3 Lasted over one year No. (%) of 1	4 Still persistent No. % of 1
Frequent headaches	419 (3.6)	368 (88)	298 (71)	263 (63)
Neckache	228 (1.9)	201 (88)	165 (72)	155 (68)
Shoulder ache	263 (2.2)	224 (85)	176 (67)	158 (59)
Ache in middle of back	719 (6.1)	633 (88)	474 (66)	441 (61)
Ache in bottom of back	1266 (10.8)	1132 (89)	905 (71)	853 (67)
Pain in arms	108 (0.9)	99 (92)	82 (76)	70 (65)
Pain in legs	240 (2.1)	210 (88)	164 (68)	145 (60)
Weakness in arms	142 (1.2)	121 (85)	94 (66)	86 (61)
Weakness in legs	148 (1.3)	129 (87)	97 (66)	86 (58)
Bowel upsets	321 (2.7)	270 (84)	206 (64)	181 (56)
Tingling in hands/fingers	293 (2.5)	260 (89)	212 (72)	192 (66)
Tingling in feet/toes	126 (1.1)	112 (89)	89 (71)	78 (62)
Buzzing in ears	76 (0.6)	69 (91)	59 (78)	55 (72)
Flashing lights/spots	174 (1.5)	157 (90)	133 (76)	117 (67)
Dizziness/fainting	211 (1.8)	172 (82)	132 (63)	117 (55)
Migraine	165 (1.4)	155 (94)	140 (85)	126 (76)
Indigestion	127 (1.1)	118 (93)	109 (86)	103 (81)
Urinary frequency	668 (5.7)	629 (94)	540 (81)	500 (75)

46

TABLE 7.2 – *continued*

Stress incontinence	1782 (15.2)	1643 (92)	1341 (75)	1246 (70)
High blood pressure	48 (0.4)	42 (88)	31 (65)	28 (58)
Haemorrhoids	931 (8.0)	786 (84)	653 (70)	621 (67)
Varicose veins	151 (1.3)	143 (95)	134 (89)	125 (83)
Dental problems	124 (1.1)	99 (80)	71 (57)	56 (45)
Depression/anxiety	1065 (9.1)	870 (82)	425 (40)	292 (27)
Extreme tiredness	1427 (12.2)	1230 (86)	717 (50)	554 (39)
Other	423 (3.6)	379 (90)	289 (68)	234 (55)
Total number of symptoms	11645	10251	7736	6882

TABLE 7.3

Onset of health problems, lasting more than six weeks and never experienced before

	1 Within 1 week No. (%) of 4	2 Within 4 weeks No. (%) of 4	3 Within 3 months No. (%) of 4	4 Within 1 year No.
Frequent headaches	221 (39)	310 (54)	419 (73)	571
Neckache	124 (38)	180 (55)	228 (70)	327
Shoulder ache	132 (36)	202 (55)	263 (71)	368
Middle backache	446 (52)	602 (70)	719 (83)	865
Lower backache	811 (52)	1033 (67)	1266 (82)	1549
Pain in arms	47 (29)	75 (46)	108 (66)	164
Pain in legs	141 (42)	184 (55)	240 (72)	334
Weakness in arms	80 (43)	106 (57)	142 (76)	186
Weakness in legs	93 (48)	120 (62)	148 (77)	193
Bowel upsets	236 (60)	274 (70)	321 (82)	391
Tingling in hands/fingers	158 (37)	208 (49)	293 (69)	424
Tingling in feet/toes	73 (44)	94 (56)	126 (75)	168
Buzzing in ears	44 (38)	56 (49)	76 (66)	115
Flashing lights/spots	84 (36)	109 (47)	174 (75)	233
Dizziness/fainting	117 (41)	151 (53)	211 (74)	287
Migraine	67 (26)	103 (39)	165 (63)	261
Indigestion	77 (43)	95 (52)	127 (70)	181
Urinary frequency	549 (76)	615 (85)	668 (93)	722
Stress incontinence	1517 (81)	1658 (89)	1782 (95)	1869
High blood pressure	35 (57)	42 (68)	48 (77)	62
Haemorrhoids	791 (79)	864 (86)	931 (93)	1002
Varicose veins	124 (65)	133 (69)	151 (78)	193
Dental problems	58 (26)	74 (33)	124 (56)	221
Depression/anxiety	587 (46)	831 (65)	1065 (83)	1286
Extreme tiredness	1039 (65)	1269 (79)	1427 (89)	1605
Other	266 (51)	316 (61)	426 (82)	520

At the other extreme only 26% of first-year dental problems and 29% of pains in the arms started in the first post-partum week. In later chapters, similar analyses for different symptoms provide useful clues in the identification of potential determinants.

Our original study objective, to identify the long-term sequelae of epidural anaesthesia, required that we focused upon symptoms starting after the delivery. The same applied to the investigation of other delivery events and procedures. In the questionnaire, we tried to make it very clear that we wanted to know whether the symptom had started **after** the baby's birth (see Appendix 1). We intended that symptoms starting during the pregnancy should not be included: symptoms that started during pregnancy even if they continued after the delivery would be categorised as 'non-first-time' symptoms. (In Table 7.1, they would be included in Column 3, but not in Column 4). However, we suspected that some women might see the whole process from the start of pregnancy to the delivery as so unified that – even with our detailed instructions – they could not separate the pregnancy from the delivery. This was probably minimal but we present evidence relating to these points for particular symptoms where there were actual indications that this might have occurred.

Medical consultation

The numbers of women who reported consulting their doctors for each type of problem are shown in Column 1 of Table 7.4. We did not ask the women how many times they had consulted with the same symptom, nor whether those with two or more symptoms had discussed both at the same consultation. These figures are based on the simplified assumption that one visit was made for each symptom.

Substantial numbers of women did not go to the doctor. The proportions who did consult varied, mostly between 30% and 40%, but there were exceptions. Among those women reporting raised blood pressure, the majority (88%) had consulted the doctor: this is not surprising since a medical examination is a general precondition to knowing that this disorder is present. Consultation rates were also relatively high for those with migraine (60%) and for the conditions (68%) reported in the open question. The label 'migraine' may also have depended selectively upon a doctor's opinion. Illnesses in the 'open' category were generally specified by name and included both 'serious' conditions and/or specifically 'labelled' conditions, those with a specific medical diagnosis; which again would account for the higher reported levels of consultation. The lowest consultation rates were for bladder problems – frequency and stress incontinence; only 22% of women with urinary frequency and 14% of those with stress incontinence went to the doctor.

TABLE 7.4

Frequency of medical consultation about health problems, treatment and referral

	1 Consulted a doctor	2 Given treatment without referral	3 Referral to hospital
	No. (%) of total with symptoms	No. (%) of 1	No. (%) of 1
Frequent headaches	201 (48)	153 (76)	13 (6)
Neckache	92 (40)	54 (59)	19 (21)
Shoulder ache	95 (36)	56 (59)	17 (18)
Middle backache	230 (32)	145 (63)	26 (11)
Lower backache	383 (30)	235 (61)	54 (14)
Pain in arms	61 (56)	33 (54)	16 (26)
Pain in legs	126 (53)	58 (46)	20 (16)
Weakness in arms	67 (47)	27 (40)	21 (31)
Weakness in legs	55 (37)	25 (45)	14 (25)
Bowel upsets	158 (49)	97 (61)	31 (20)
Tingling in hands/fingers	113 (39)	33 (29)	35 (31)
Tingling in feet/toes	57 (45)	14 (25)	17 (30)
Buzzing in ears	31 (41)	13 (42)	7 (23)
Flashing lights/spots	60 (34)	37 (62)	10 (17)
Dizziness/fainting	105 (50)	57 (54)	15 (14)
Migraine	99 (60)	83 (84)	5 (5)
Indigestion	50 (39)	35 (70)	9 (18)
Urinary frequency	149 (22)	63 (42)	47 (32)
Stress incontinence	242 (14)	121 (50)	61 (25)
High blood pressure	42 (88)	27 (64)	2 (5)
Haemorrhoids	415 (45)	359 (87)	23 (6)
Varicose veins	59 (39)	16 (27)	23 (39)
Dental problems	107 (86)	N/A	N/A
Depression/anxiety	514 (48)	310 (60)	54 (11)
Extreme tiredness	373 (26)	198 (53)	37 (10)
Other	286 (68)	155 (54)	67 (23)
Total no. of symptoms	4170	2404	643

The severity of a condition may in part determine whether a woman consults her doctor. The relationship however is not straightforward and a woman's decision whether or not to visit will depend on other factors as well. Perceptions as to which symptoms are appropriate to take to a doctor will vary, as will symptoms regarded by some women as 'normal'. Particular women, according to their age, race, social class, etc., may be more or less likely than others to consult the doctor, and these patterns will vary for different symptoms. Different patterns of consulting for specific symptoms are described in later chapters.

An independent measure of the severity of each symptom would have been useful in these analyses but it would have been difficult to obtain information of this nature about so many complaints in this type of enquiry. This demands a different approach and must remain for the present a subject for further investigation.

Treatment

We included a question for each symptom enquiring about the type of treatment (if any) that the doctor had given. We were only able to categorise this very generally since many women reported, for example, only that 'he gave me some tablets', or, 'I got some cream'. Only infrequently would the woman give the name of the preparation. In view of this problem we have tabulated (Table 7.4) just the total numbers and proportions who had treatment of any kind from the general practitioner (Column 2); and those who said they were referred for specialist investigation and/or treatment (Column 3). This latter category includes those who had surgery, those who consulted but had other forms of treatment, as well as those who had hospital outpatient investigations but no recorded treatment. Again, some women were specific about the details but others answered with responses such as 'he sent me to the hospital' or even just 'hospital'. The question on treatment did not specifically ask about referral to the hospital, and some women will have omitted to tell us about referrals for investigations or consultations where treatment was not given.

Of the women consulting their general practitioner the proportion who were given treatment varied considerably for the different symptoms. It was as high as 87% for piles, 84% for migraine and 76% for frequent headaches; while much lower proportions received treatment from the general practitioner for tingling in the feet (25%) or hands (29%) and varicose veins (27%). The proportions referred also differed greatly, with very low referrals for high blood pressure (5%) migraine (5%), headaches (6%) and haemorrhoids (6%); while 39% of women consulting with varicose veins were referred, 32% with urinary frequency and 31% and 30% for tingling in the hands or feet. High rates of general practitioner treatment rates were directly related to low referral rates.

Over the whole range of post-partum symptoms the frequency of specialist referral was low. The total of 643 symptoms referred, comprised only 5.5% of all those reported and defined by us as relevant to the index delivery (Table 7.1, Column 4).

Total number of symptoms

So far we have described only the numbers and proportions of women reporting with individual symptoms, but we have not yet described the average load per woman, or the manner in which this load was distributed. In Tables 7.1 and 7.2, at the foot of each column, we have shown the total number of symptoms reported according to each of the different criteria. According to our final symptom-relevance criteria, i.e. first time symptoms occurring within three

TABLE 7.5

Number of all health problems and number that were persistent, reported by each woman

Number of symptoms	All Symptoms*			Persistent Symptoms**	
	Total women	% of sample (11701)	% of those reporting symptoms (5457)	Total women	% of sample (11701)
None	6244	53.4	–	8016	68.5
One	2546	21.8	46.7	2075	17.1
Two	1435	12.3	26.3	899	7.7
Three	703	6.0	12.9	347	3.0
Four	376	3.2	6.9	179	1.5
Five	169	1.4	3.1	77	0.7
Six	82	0.7	1.5	39	0.3
Seven	62	0.5	1.1	26	0.2
Eight	32	0.3	0.6	13	0.1
Nine	16	0.1	0.3	12	0.1
Ten	11	0.1	0.2	3	0.03
Eleven or more	25	0.2	0.5	15	0.1

*First time occurrences within three months of delivery and lasting more than six weeks

**First time occurrences within three months of delivery and still present at the time of questioning

months of delivery, and lasting more than six weeks (Table 7.1., Column 4), the total amounted to 11,645 reports. This represents a mean of about one symptom per woman. However, 6244 women reported no such symptoms; among the remaining 5457 women the mean number was 2.1. Table 7.5 gives a full distribution of the numbers of symptoms each woman had reported. Most women who reported any symptoms, reported only one (47%) or two (26%): but 13% reported three; 7% reported four, and 7% reported more than four.

Table 7.5 (Panel 2) also gives the numbers of women who reported one or more symptoms which were still present at the time of our enquiry. A total of 3685 women (31.5% of the sample) said that at least one of their symptoms, starting for the first time within three months of the delivery, had still not subsided. Of these 3685, most (56.3%) had only one persisting complaint, but 24.4% had two; 9.4% had three; and 9.9% had more than three unresolved symptoms.

Year of index delivery and symptom persistence

Some of the women included in the investigation had delivered their babies nine years earlier, while for others this was only thirteen months. This variation could have two main effects upon our analyses. First, the year of delivery could influence a woman's recollection of her health problems. A symptom which had lasted even for several months could be forgotten if it had occurred several years before; or its associations could have been confused with another delivery. Second, short intervals since delivery truncate the record of the symptom's natural history, and restrict any assessments of chronicity made at the time of the enquiry. It is also possible that standards of obstetric practice could have changed and that the incidence of certain symptoms could have declined or increased.

In Chapter 4 we reported that the proportions of women reporting symptoms did indeed vary according to the year of delivery. We concluded that there must be some under-reporting of symptoms in women who had their babies several years before and that the real morbidity rates were probably higher than those reported. The full details of morbidity levels according to year of birth are supplied now in Table 7.6 and shown graphically in Fig 7.4. The gradient is clear, although the differences are generally quite small. Overall, among women who had delivered in 1978 and 1979, 38% reported at least one symptom, compared with 51% of those who had delivered in 1984 or 1985. The corresponding mean numbers of symptoms per woman were 0.77 and 1.11 respectively.

We also examined the persistence of symptoms in women delivering in the earlier and in the later years. The continued presence of a symptom thirteen

TABLE 7.6

Proportion of women reporting health problems according to year of delivery

	1978-79 (n = 1401)	1980-81 (n = 1974)	1982-83 (n = 3207)	1984-85 (n = 5119)
Frequent headaches	31 (2.2)	59 (3.0)	99 (3.1)	223 (4.4)
Neckache	24 (1.7)	34 (1.7)	58 (1.8)	112 (2.2)
Shoulder ache	19 (1.4)	37 (1.9)	67 (2.1)	140 (2.7)
Middle backache	49 (3.5)	82 (4.2)	192 (6.0)	396 (7.7)
Lower backache	114 (8.1)	187 (9.5)	332 (10.4)	633 (12.4)
Pain in arms	7 (0.5)	15 (0.8)	27 (0.8)	59 (1.2)
Pain in legs	15 (1.1)	37 (1.9)	68 (2.1)	120 (2.3)
Weakness in arms	9 (0.6)	18 (0.9)	29 (0.9)	86 (1.7)
Weakness in legs	8 (0.6)	21 (1.1)	40 (1.2)	79 (1.5)
Bowel upsets	33 (2.4)	43 (2.2)	78 (2.4)	166 (3.2)
Tingling in hands/fingers	26 (1.9)	50 (2.5)	75 (2.3)	142 (2.8)
Tingling in feet/toes	13 (0.9)	22 (1.1)	29 (0.9)	61 (1.2)
Buzzing in ears	7 (0.5)	9 (0.5)	23 (0.7)	37 (0.7)
Visual disturbances	14 (1.0)	30 (1.5)	46 (1.4)	84 (1.6)
Dizziness/fainting	15 (1.0)	32 (1.6)	53 (1.7)	111 (2.2)
Migraine	26 (1.9)	28 (1.4)	37 (1.2)	74 (1.4)
Indigestion	14 (1.0)	26 (1.3)	42 (1.3)	47 (0.9)
Urinary frequency	69 (4.9)	111 (5.6)	193 (6.0)	295 (5.8)
Stress incontinence	171 (12.2)	268 (13.4)	511 (15.9)	836 (16.3)
High blood pressure	8 (0.6)	7 (0.4)	9 (0.3)	20 (0.4)
Haemorrhoids	103 (7.4)	140 (7.1)	275 (8.6)	413 (8.1)
Varicose veins	30 (2.1)	27 (1.4)	41 (1.3)	53 (1.0)
Dental problems	13 (0.9)	17 (0.9)	33 (1.0)	61 (1.2)
Depression/anxiety	115 (8.2)	164 (8.3)	290 (9.0)	496 (9.7)
Extreme tiredness	115 (8.2)	196 (9.9)	375 (11.8)	739 (14.4)
Other	34 (2.4)	62 (3.1)	121 (3.8)	206 (4.0)
Total symptoms	1082	1722	3143	5689
Mean per woman	0.77	0.87	0.98	1.11
Prop. of women reporting at least one symptom	38.3	40.6	46.8	51.2

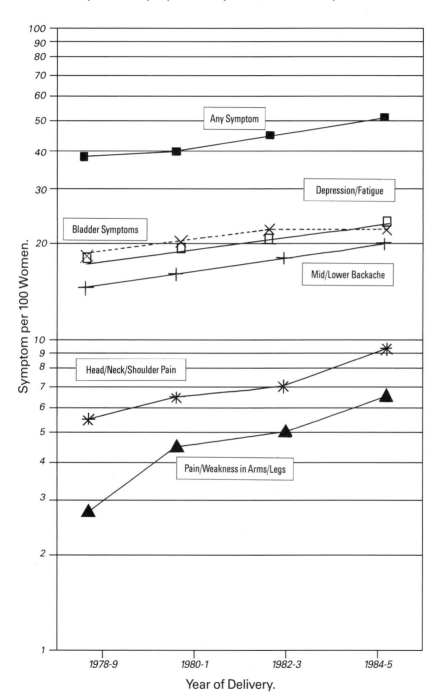

Figure 7.4
Reported Symptoms by Year of Delivery

TABLE 7.7

Proportion of women who reported persistence of health problems and year of delivery

	Number with persistent symptoms (%) of total with symptoms for those years	
	1978-81 deliveries	1982-85 deliveries
Frequent headaches	60 (62)	203 (63)
Neckache	41 (71)	114 (67)
Shoulder ache	37 (66)	121 (58)
Middle backache	80 (61)	361 (61)
Lower backache	212 (70)	641 (66)
Pain in arms	16 (73)	54 (63)
Pain in legs	38 (73)	107 (57)
Weakness in arms	17 (63)	69 (60)
Weakness in legs	20 (69)	69 (58)
Bowel upsets	48 (62)	133 (55)
Tingling in hands/fingers	50 (66)	142 (65)
Tingling in feet/toes	22 (61)	56 (62)
Buzzing in ears	14 (88)	41 (68)
Visual disturbances	29 (66)	88 (68)
Dizziness/fainting	30 (64)	87 (53)
Migraine	46 (85)	80 (72)
Indigestion	31 (82)	72 (81)
Urinary frequency	140 (78)	360 (74)
Stress incontinence	350 (80)*	896 (67)
High blood pressure	12 (80)	16 (53)
Haemorrhoids	178 (73)*	443 (64)
Varicose veins	44 (77)	81 (86)
Dental problems	9 (30)	47 (50)
Depression/anxiety	68 (24)	224 (28)
Extreme tiredness	107 (34)	447 (40)
Other	51 (53)	183 (56)

* See text

months after childbirth does not in itself imply that it has become permanent: although if several years have elapsed it might justifiably be labelled as chronic. In Table 7.7 the proportions still complaining of symptoms at the time of the enquiry are compared in women who had delivered within five years (1982-85), and in those who had delivered five years or more before the questions were posed (1978-81). In fact there were few differences. This implies that many symptoms which had lasted for one to five years, had by then become permanent. The last two columns of Table 7.2 show in fact that the majority of symptoms lasting for more than a year (Column 3), were still present (Column 4). Once these conditions were established to this extent, there was little evidence of recovery as the years passed.

Only for two conditions were there significant differences according to the year of delivery. They were stress incontinence and haemorrhoids. Both displayed a greater reported prevalence of persistent symptoms following deliveries in the **earlier** years. This is the reverse of that expected from a declining rate of recall with the passage of time. We show in later chapters that these two symptoms are closely related to pelvic trauma during delivery. The difference might therefore represent genuine changes in obstetric practice, with a decreasing risk for more recent deliveries.

Discussion

This chapter supplies the first substantive results of our investigation. Our enquiries have revealed an enormous and previously unrecognised problem: a level of post-partum morbidity and impaired health far beyond anything which might have been suspected. These women suffered a wide range of different symptoms, many of which had become chronic, resulting in a high prevalence of long-term health problems. Many of the women for whatever reason did not seek medical help.

We must not assume that every one of these new health problems that started within the post-partum three months, and lasted for more than six weeks, was related directly to the delivery of the index child. Many changes occur after childbirth that are more specifically related to caring for a child, and some will be associated with the listed symptoms. Some symptoms starting during the three post-partum months may be entirely urelated either to childbirth or to child care. We considered recruiting a group of women without children as comparisons, but realised that childlesss women are different in so many other ways. And for the purposes of identifying the potential determinants of symptoms we had internal control groups: the women who had not had a particular obstetric procedure or who were from a different social group. The childbirth-specificities of the different symptoms are discussed later in relation to the individual health problems.

Each of the following chapters describes a specific health problem or set of problems in much greater detail, seeking to identify their potential social, obstetric or anaesthetic determinants. We commence with the most frequent ones.

Chapter 8 – Backache

Two questions about backache were included in the questionnaire on post-partum health problems. Since the delivery of her child, had the women had 'ache in the middle of the back?': and had she had 'ache in the bottom of the back?'.

Frequency of occurrence

For those symptoms which began within three months of the nominated delivery, lasted for more than six weeks, and had never occurred before: 368 (3.1%) women reported middle backache; 915 (7.8%) reported lower backache; and another 351 (3%) reported both. In all, this amounted to 1634 women (14%).

A further 1096 (9%) women reported backache (lasting over six weeks and occurring within three months of delivery) but which they had also had previously. This brings the total up to 2730 (23.4%), of whom 60% had this symptom for the first time. Among the primiparous women, 72% of the backaches were 'first-time' compared with 51% in multiparae, suggesting that some of the previous backaches reported by the multiparous women must have been associated specifically with earlier births.

Other women – 336 with middle backache and 576 with lower backache – did not provide the exact dates of their symptom. All of them said that the problem had occurred at some time since the index delivery, but they did not give the time of onset, or the duration, or say whether it was newly occurring. These inadequately dated reports were excluded from the above prevalence estimates which we must therefore regard as minima. They were also excluded from the analyses which we report below.

The main analyses in this chapter are based upon the 1634 women who had accurately dated backache, starting for the first time within three months of the birth, and lasting more than six weeks. The purpose of the 'first time' restriction was to maximise the specificity of correlation between the backache and the events associated with the nominated birth. Initially we conducted analyses for middle and lower backache separately and these are shown in some of the Tables; but the differences were never substantial. Because of this, and because it is anyway difficult in a postal questionnaire to be precise about the exact anatomical location, we subsequently aggregated middle and lower backache within a single group.

Durations and onsets

All 1634 cases of backache had persisted for more than six weeks, but most had lasted much longer than this. Only 10% had gone within three months and 70%

lasted for more than a year. For 65% the backache was still present at the time of our enquiry.

All 1634 backaches had begun within the first three post-partum months, but most (63% – 1028) started within a week of the delivery, and 82% (1341) within four weeks. The remaining 293 began in the second or third months.

Although excluded from our main analyses, another 357 women reported newly occurring and persistent backaches beginning between three and twelve months after the delivery, making an overall total of 1991 within the first year. If backaches had been unrelated to delivery we would expect them to be evenly distributed throughout the year, but 52% of first-year backaches commenced within the first week, 67% within four weeks and 82% within three months of delivery. This indicates that although backache is not exclusively childbirth-specific, many cases are related in some way to the delivery of a child.

Medical consultation

Despite the lengthy durations of most backaches, only 30% of affected women had consulted a doctor. Combined middle and lower backache had a higher consulting rate, 41%: joint reporting might have indicated a greater severity. For those with only middle or only lower backache the proportions consulting were 26% and 27% respectively. However, neither the duration nor the continued persistence of the backache (middle, lower or both) provoked an increase in medical consultations. We might perhaps have expected that more of the women with persistent backache would have consulted: but we have no direct information on the reasons for non-consultation.

The only social or demographic characteristic which seemed to influence the likelihood of a medical consultation, was ethnic group. Asian women with backache were more likely to consult a doctor than were the other races. They also had more backache, as we shall see below.

We asked the women about treatment for their backache. Of those who went to the doctor, 61% said that they had received some form of treatment; 40% reported receiving tablets, the remaining 21% other treatments (e.g. physiotherapy), while 13% said they had been referred to the hospital. Women reporting both middle and lower backache were not more likely either to be treated or to be referred.

Factors associated with backache

Simple statistical associations between backache, and the various social obstetric and anaesthetic factors are shown in Table 8.1 and demonstrated graphically in Figure 8.1. Associations with the social and demographic

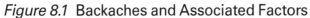

Figure 8.1 Backaches and Associated Factors

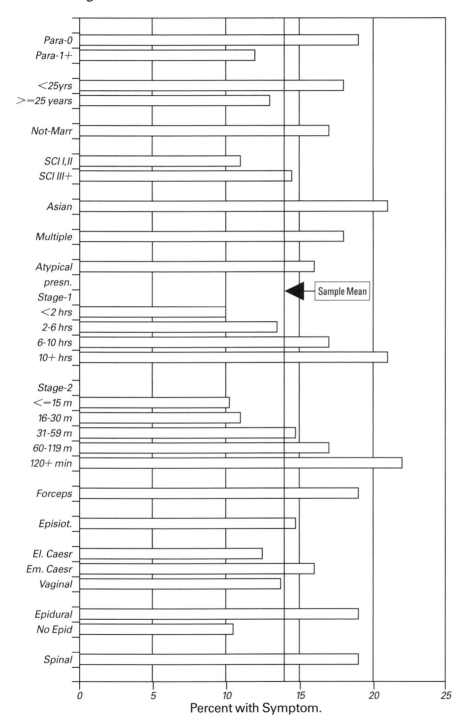

Percent with Symptom.

TABLE 8.1

Characteristics associated with backache*

	Just Middle No. (%)	Just Lower No. (%)	Both No. (%)	Total with backache No. (%)	Total women
Whole sample	368 (3.1)	915 (7.8)	351 (3.0)	1634 (14.0)	11701
Primiparae	188 (4.5)	403 (9.6)	199 (4.8)	790 (18.9)	4185
Multiparae	180 (2.4)	512 (6.8)	152 (2.0)	844 (11.2)	7516
Under 25 years	107 (4.1)	237 (9.0)	125 (4.8)	469 (17.9)	2625
25 or more	261 (2.9)	678 (7.5)	226 (2.5)	1165 (12.8)	9076
Married	326 (3.1)	811 (7.7)	294 (2.8)	1431 (13.6)	10525
Single/Div/Wid/Sep	42 (3.6)	104 (8.8)	56 (4.8)	202 (17.2)	1176
Social Class					
I and II	89 (3.1)	190 (6.6)	50 (1.7)	329 (11.4)	2882
III, IV & V	215 (3.0)	559 (7.9)	226 (3.2)	1000 (14.2)	7050
Caucasian	302 (3.0)	808 (8.0)	284 (2.8)	1394 (13.8)	10135
Asian	32 (6.0)	42 (7.9)	39 (7.4)	113 (21.3)	530
Singleton	363 (3.1)	896 (7.8)	344 (3.0)	1603 (13.9)	11532
Multiple	5 (3.0)	19 (11.2)	7 (4.1)	31 (18.3)	169
Occipito-Anterior	322 (3.1)	786 (7.7)	299 (2.9)	1407 (13.7)	10265
Other presentations	46 (3.2)	129 (9.0)	52 (3.6)	227 (15.9)	1430
First stage labour					
Under 2 hours	47 (2.3)	125 (6.1)	33 (1.6)	205 (10.0)	2054
2 – 5 hrs 59 mins	157 (3.0)	408 (7.8)	152 (2.9)	717 (13.6)	5264
6 – 9 hrs 59 mins	57 (3.4)	169 (10.0)	63 (3.7)	289 (17.2)	1684
10 hours or more	22 (4.3)	59 (11.5)	25 (4.9)	106 (20.7)	511

characteristics of the mothers, are shown in the upper part of Table 8.1. There were distinct differences according to parity, age, marital status, and ethnic group.

Primiparous women were most likely to report post-partum backache: 18.9% compared with 11.2% in multiparae. It was also reported more frequently by younger women: 17.9% of mothers under 25 compared with 12.8% of those aged 25 years or more. These findings are inter-related in two ways. First, younger

TABLE 8.1 – *continued*

	Just Middle No. (%)	Just Lower No. (%)	Both No. (%)	Total with backache No. (%)	Total women
Second stage labour					
Up to 15 minutes	75 (2.5)	184 (6.1)	48 (1.6)	307 (10.2)	3014
16 – 30 minutes	48 (2.2)	142 (6.6)	50 (2.3)	240 (11.2)	2142
31 – 59 minutes	54 (3.1)	139 (7.9)	65 (3.7)	258 (14.8)	1749
60 – 119 minutes	66 (3.8)	199 (10.7)	69 (3.7)	334 (18.0)	1858
120 minutes or more	49 (5.2)	112 (11.9)	45 (4.8)	20 (21.9)	939
Forceps	89 (3.9)	235 (10.2)	105 (4.6)	429 (18.6)	2301
No forceps	279 (3.0)	680 (7.2)	246 (2.6)	1205 (12.8)	9400
Episiotomy	161 (3.1)	430 (8.4)	173 (3.4)	764 (14.9)	5112
No episiotomy	207 (3.1)	485 (7.4)	178 (2.7)	870 (13.2)	6589
Elective section	22 (2.9)	51 (6.6)	24 (3.1)	97 (12.6)	770
Emergency section	49 (4.3)	86 (7.5)	52 (4.5)	187 (16.3)	1145
Vaginal delivery	297 (3.0)	778 (7.9)	275 (2.8)	1350 (13.8)	9786
Epidural	193 (4.0)	503 (10.6)	207 (4.3)	903 (18.9)	4766
No epidural	175 (2.5)	412 (5.9)	144 (2.1)	731 (10.5)	6935
Spinal anaesthesia	6 (3.8)	16 (10.0)	9 (5.6)	31 (19.4)	160
No spinal anaesthesia	362 (3.1)	899 (7.8)	342 (3.0)	1603 (13.9)	11541

*Backaches starting within three months of delivery, never previously experienced, lasting longer than six weeks.

women were more likely to be having a first baby. Second, the exclusion of non-first-time backaches would act selectively upon older affected women, and upon multiparae.

Unmarried women reported a higher prevalence of backache (17.2%) than married women (13.6%), and women in social classes I and II had less (11.4%) than those in other social classes (14.2%). Both findings could be secondary to the relationship with parity, since unmarried women and those in the higher social classes had fewer previous children.

Asian women, of whom 93% were Indian or Pakistani, were much more likely to report backache than were the other races. Of the 530 Asian women in the sample, 113 (21.3%) reported this symptom. The relative risk of such backache among Asian women was 1.54, compared with the Caucasian women. This excess was not secondary to a primiparity effect, since in this particular sample the first-birth proportion among the Asian women did **not** differ, as is typically the case, from the Caucasians.

The statistical correlations of backache with the obstetric circumstances of the delivery, and with the obstetric and anaesthetic procedures employed, are given in the lower part of Table 8.1, and again there were several clear associations.

Women who had a multiple pregnancy or an atypical fetal presentation reported more backache than did normal singletons. There was a systematic linear association between the duration of labour and rates of backache. This was present, and in the same direction, for both first and second stages. Only 7.2% of women with a first stage lasting under one hour reported backache compared with three times as many (20.7%) where first stage lasted ten hours or more. Similarly, only 9.2% of those with a second stage of five minutes or less reported backache, compared with 23.6% of those with a second stage of three hours or more. The durations of the two stages of labour are themselves positively correlated with each other (see Chapter 6), and both are related to numerous other factors, for example parity, multiple pregnancy, abnormal presentations and epidural anaesthesia.

Backache was also associated with several specific obstetric and anaesthetic procedures. There were positive associations with forceps delivery, emergency Caesarean section, epidural anaesthesia, spinal anaesthesia, and episiotomy. Again, several of these factors were associated with each other, as well as with the durations of the stages of labour (above), and with some of the social and demographic factors. The other forms of analgesia and anaesthesia were not associated with backache; nor was induction of labour, nor the length of gestation at delivery, nor the baby's birthweight or head circumference or length.

Primary predictors and secondary associations

From among all the social and obstetric factors associated with backache, we needed to separate the primary independent correlations from those which were more probably secondary. To do this we used the statistical technique of discriminant analysis, which takes simultaneous account of all factors before identifying those which act as primary independent predictors. The results are shown in Table 8.2. The first two columns of Table 8.2 relate to vaginal

TABLE 8.2

Discriminant analysis of characteristics associated with backache

| | Vaginal deliveries | | All deliveries | |
	F-value	Coefficients	F-value	Coefficients
Epidural	83.789	0.63002	142.97	0.75063
Primaparity	29.688	0.38387	46.608	0.41497
Asian ethnic group	23.392	0.28261	21.345	0.25525
Younger age	16.07	0.25584	22.438	0.28264
No episiotomy	9.9692	0.20784	5.6348	0.13561
Longer 2nd stage labour	6.4389	0.18714	N/A	N/A
Spinal anaesthesia	7.7306	0.16456	7.4467	0.15192
Non-induced labour	5.267	0.13683	5.5317	0.13221
Social class III, IV, V	4.0318	0.12054	5.7251	0.13883

deliveries only: the last two columns to all types of delivery. The analysis in the first two columns (but not in the last two) incorporated duration of labour as predictor-variables. The analysis shown in the last two columns included Caesarean sections – for which durations of labour were not recorded. The factors shown to be independent predictors of backache were epidural anaesthesia, primiparity, Asian ethnic group, early maternal age, a longer second stage of labour, spinal anaesthesia and lower social class. Episiotomy and induced labour showed negative associations. Epidural anaesthesia showed by far the most highly significant association and the largest discriminant co-efficient, within each of the two analyses.

All of these predictors were then examined further by constructing multi-way tabulations relating each of them to backache and to the other predictors. From this we hoped to move towards a more confident identification of the potential determinants of post-partum backache.

Social predictors

Among the mothers' social and demographic characteristics, parity appeared from the discriminant analysis to be the dominant independent predictor, with younger maternal age, Asian ethnic group and (to a lesser extent) lower social class (III, IV, V), retaining additional independent effects.

Parity and age

The relationships with parity and maternal age probably arose in part from limiting the investigation to 'first time' backaches, selectively excluding a greater proportion of affected multiparae and older women. If (as our data show) 18.9% of primiparous women get newly occurring long-term backache, then only 81.1% of the women delivering a second child, would be 'at risk' of having 'first-time' backache after this second delivery. For third and fourth deliveries the proportions of eligible respondents are progressively reduced as the numbers of women without previous backache diminish. These same parity/age considerations will apply to other symptoms and disorders examined in later chapters.

In order to clarify this issue further, we conducted a subsidiary discriminant analysis, this time including **all** the post-delivery longer-term backaches (2730), **irrespective** of whether they were first-time or not. Here, the association with primiparity disappeared and the association with age was much diminished. This tends to confirm our interpretation. That is, the reduced rates of backache reported after later births are unlikely to be real, and the apparent excess in younger women is spurious. The effects of social class likewise disappeared, suggesting that this association was also secondary to parity.

Ethnic group

Although the associations of backache with primiparity, younger age and lower social class were largely artefacts, the Asian association was not. The excess of backache among Asian women compared with Caucasian women remained highly significant irrespective of whether or not we included non-first-time backaches, and irrespective of the obstetric procedures employed. We discuss this further later.

Obstetric and anaesthetic predictors

The independent associations with the different obstetric and anaesthetic procedures, and the circumstances of the delivery, are shown in Table 8.2, the main independent obstetric predictors of backache being epidural anaesthesia, a longer second stage labour and spinal anaesthesia. The initial statistical associations with multiple pregnancy, fetal presentation and forceps delivery had all disappeared as secondary associations. The crude association with the duration of first stage labour was also dispersed; the duration of second stage appeared as the primary predictor. Episiotomy and induced labour were negatively associated with backache. But of all the independent predictors of backache, epidural anaesthesia was much the most powerful. Furthermore, as we discuss below, the association between backache and epidural anaesthesia was confirmed consistently both in simple and in multivariate analyses and in a range of different sub-tabulations.

Epidural anaesthesia

Overall, backache occurred in 18.9% of women who had epidural anaesthesia compared with 10.5% of those who did not. The crude relative risk was 1.80. Among the relatively small number of women receiving spinal anaesthesia (160), a similar proportion (19.4%) of women had subsequent backache.

This powerful association between backache and epidural anaesthesia was unexpected. We considered whether there might still be an indirect explanation. It is well known that epidural anaesthesia is more frequently given in 'abnormal' or 'difficult' pre-delivery circumstances (e.g. atypical fetal presentation), and is associated with less straightforward deliveries (e.g. long second stage, forceps). Despite the standardisation effected through the discriminant analysis, we needed to be sure that the association did not result from complex non-linear relationships between these different factors. We therefore re-assembled the evidence to show whether the epidural association with backache was consistently visible within a wide range of separate sub-groups.

Epidural anaesthesia and 'normal' deliveries

First, we defined a group of women who had 'normal' or straightforward deliveries. A 'normal' delivery was defined for these purposes as a singleton with an occipito-anterior presentation, a spontaneous onset of labour, no forceps, no Caesarean section, a first stage of labour of less than twelve hours and a second stage of less than two hours. The 'abnormals' were the remainder. The association between epidurals and backache was then tested in each group separately.

Table 8.3 presents the frequencies of backache in the four classes of women: 'normal' and 'abnormal' deliveries, with and without epidural. The relationships are demonstrated graphically in Figure 8.2. An epidural was associated with a higher rate of subsequent backache both in normal and in abnormal deliveries. Furthermore, an abnormal delivery was not in fact associated with a raised risk of subsequent backache. The overall relative risk of having backache after an epidural, taking no account of the normality of

TABLE 8.3

Backache, epidural anaesthesia and 'normal' deliveries

	Just Middle No. (%)	Just Lower No. (%)	Both No. (%)	Total with backache No. (%)	Total women
'Normal' delivery with epidural	40 (3.6)	118 (10.7)	42 (3.8)	200 (18.2)	1098
'Normal' delivery: no epidural	112 (2.4)	280 (6.0)	82 (1.8)	474 (10.2)	4646
'Abnormal' delivery with epidural	153 (4.2)	385 (10.5)	165 (4.5)	703 (19.2)	3668
'Abnormal' delivery, no epidural	63 (2.8)	132 (5.8)	62 (2.7)	257 (11.2)	2289

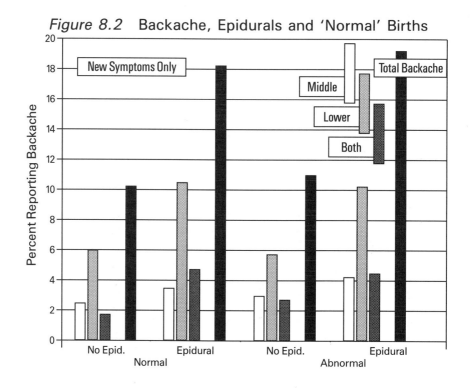

Figure 8.2   Backache, Epidurals and 'Normal' Births

TABLE 8.4

Backache, epidural anaesthesia and second stage of labour

Duration of 2nd stage	No Epidural		Epidural	
	Backache No. (%)	Total women	Backache No. (%)	Total women
Up to 5 mins	45 (8.3)	542	9 (17.6)	51
6 – 10	108 (9.3)	1160	20 (16.1)	124
11 – 15	97 (10.2)	954	28 (15.3)	183
16 – 30	143 (9.0)	1594	97 (17.7)	548
31 – 59	116 (11.6)	999	142 (19.0)	749
60 – 90	66 (14.7)	448	130 (18.8)	691
91 – 119	30 (15.0)	200	108 (20.8)	519
120 – 179	25 (24.8)	101	133 (20.9)	636
180 mins or more	—	13	47 (24.7)	190

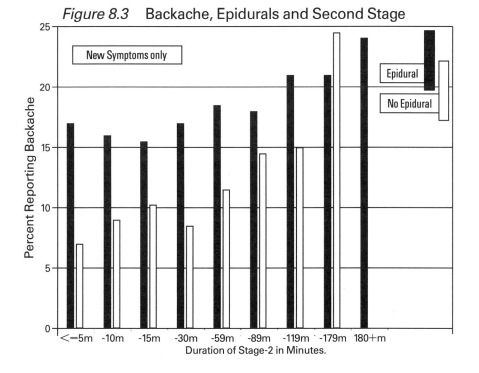

Figure 8.3   Backache, Epidurals and Second Stage

delivery, was 1.80. Among the 'normal' deliveries it was 1.79 and among the 'abnormals' it was 1.71. There was nothing here to cast doubt on the precedence and power of the epidural relationship with backache, as displayed in the discriminant procedure. Even though this analysis showed clearly that the 'abnormal' deliveries did have a much higher usage of epidural, 62% compared with 19% among the 'normals' (Table 8.3), we could not account for the excess backache after an epidural, through this route.

Epidural anaesthesia and duration of second stage labour

Longer second stage labour showed an independent positive association with backache, although a long second stage was also correlated with epidural anaesthesia. We therefore examined the interactions between epidurals and second stage durations in more detail (Table 8.4 and Figure 8.3). This showed that backache rates rose as the duration of the second stage lengthened, both in epidural and in non-epidural deliveries, but the gradient was steeper among the non-epidural deliveries, and the relative effect of an epidural was greater in the short labours. Although a longer second stage was associated with increased backache independently of epidural anaesthesia, the differences were greater in the absence of an epidural. This suggests that epidural anaesthesia, and a long second stage, to some extent might reflect alternative rather than synergistic pathways towards postpartum backache.

Epidural and spinal anaesthesia

Epidural and spinal anaesthesias are in some respects similar, and were mutually exclusive in practice, but the latter was used in only 160 deliveries. It was most frequently used for forceps deliveries, especially rotational forceps: 65% of the women with spinal anaesthesia had forceps, compared with a forceps rate of 19.7% in the total sample. Correspondingly, many spinal anaesthesias (38%) were associated with a second stage labour of more than two hours, compared with only 8% in the total population. Only ten spinal blocks were used for Caesarean section: a matter of policy at that time. The main differences between spinal and epidural anaesthesia are that the former is a single shot procedure followed by withdrawal of the needle and was almost always given during second stage, being of relatively short duration, generally lasting about 1-2 hours. Yet its backache-relationship was similar to that of epidurals. This offered some clues about the possible mechanisms of causation, as we discuss later.

Epidural anaesthesia and Caesarean section

Next, we examined elective and emergency Caesarean sections and compared them with vaginal deliveries. The two types of section are used in different circumstances and, in particular, women with elective sections have no labour. Table 8.5 and Figure 8.4 show that similar proportions of women delivering by elective and by emergency sections (55% and 57%) had epidural anaesthesia. This was greater than for vaginal deliveries, where epidural usage was 38%. The relative risk of backache following an epidural was similar among the emergency sections (1.77) and vaginal deliveries (1.86); but for elective Caesarean section the picture was quite different.

Elective sections without epidural had the same rate of subsequent backache as did emergency sections without epidural and the non-epidural vaginal deliveries. However, an epidural in women having elective sections was not associated with subsequent backache; the rate was **not** significantly increased after this type of delivery. This finding is of great importance in considering possible causal mechanisms of backache, and we shall return to this point later.

Women who had an emergency Caesarean section and epidural anaesthesia could be subdivided further; some (42%) had an epidural for pain relief during labour but went on to have a general anaesthetic for the Caesarean section itself, whilst the remainder (58%) had the operation under epidural block. Nevertheless the rates of backache in these different circumstances were enhanced equally to 19.9% and 20.3% respectively.

In summary then, these detailed examinations of different types of delivery confirmed the pre-eminence of epidural anaesthesia as the most powerful predictor of backache. But the relationship was not present in elective sections. It was limited only to women who had undergone a period in labour.

Epidural anaesthesia and pain tolerance

One major potential artefact remains to be considered: the possible relationship between individual tolerance of pain and the choice of pain relief during labour. Suppose that some women choose to have an epidural because they have a low pain threshold or a low pain tolerance; either they are less able to withstand pain or they are more likely to complain of it. If such pain intolerance contributed jointly to the likelihood of choosing an epidural and of reporting subsequent back pain, then the observed association might reflect nothing more than a correlated propensity to complain of pain on separate occasions.

There was no explicit record in the case notes as to why different women had their epidurals. The notes did not show whether they made the choice

TABLE 8.5

Backache, epidural anaesthesia and type of delivery

	Backache No. (%)	Total women
Elective with epidural	59 (13.8)	426
Elective, no epidural	38 (11.0)	344
Emergency with epidural	131 (20.0)	652
Emergency, no epidural	56 (11.3)	493
Vaginal with epidural	713 (19.3)	3688
Vaginal, no epidural	637 (10.4)	6098

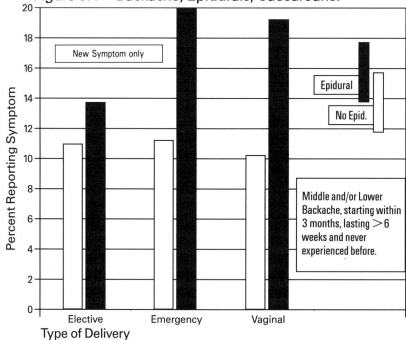

Figure 8.4 Backache, Epidurals, Caesareans.

New Symptom only

Epidural

No Epid.

Middle and/or Lower Backache, starting within 3 months, lasting >6 weeks and never experienced before.

Percent Reporting Symptom

Type of Delivery

Elective   Emergency   Vaginal

themselves and asked for the procedure, or whether it was advised, perhaps because of obstetric indications. However, we identified a number of pre-delivery obstetric circumstances which on prior grounds seemed more likely to result in such advice. They were maternal hypertension, an induced labour, an atypical fetal presentation, or a multiple birth. We then showed that the epidural rates were indeed greater when these conditions were recorded. Among the 2241 women with vaginal deliveries where at least one of these indications was present, 59% had an epidural, compared with an epidural rate of 31% among the 7545 vaginal deliveries with none of these indications. Other things being equal, we would expect a greater proportion of 'low pain tolerance' requests for an epidural among the 'no-indication' epidurals; and if the pain tolerance hypothesis was correct, there should have been a greater post-epidural reporting-rate of backache in this group. In fact, there was no difference between the groups. Because of the parity differences of backache, we tabulated the relationship for primiparae and multiparae separately. Among the primiparae, 21.3% of the 'indication' epidurals reported backache, compared with 25% of the 'no-indication' epidurals. Among the multiparae, backache rates were 14.1% in the 'indication' epidurals and 15.7% in the 'no indication' epidurals. There was no evidence here that the association between epidurals and subsequent backache could be explained by the existence of a group of persistent complainers.

Epidural anaesthesia and Asian ethnic group

Asian ethnic group was a powerful independent predictor of backache. We examined this in connection with epidural anaesthesia. Table 8.6 and Figure 8.5 show that with or without an epidural, Asian women had significantly increased rates of backache compared with Caucasian women. Second, it showed that epidurals had an additional effect as powerful as among the Caucasians. The effects were additive. Asian women who had an epidural reported subsequent backache rates of 30.2%.

Epidural anaesthesia, induction and episiotomy

Discriminant analysis demonstrated independent negative associations between backache on the one hand and induced deliveries and episiotomies, on the other. Tabulations for epidural and non-epidural deliveries separately (Tables 8.7 and 8.8) showed that the reduced rates of backache associated with induced labours and episiotomy only occurred in the presence of an epidural. These associations were relatively weak and it is difficult to think of an explanation.

TABLE 8.6

Backache, epidural anaesthesia and Asian ethnic group

	Backache No. (%)	Total women
Asian, with epidural	61 (30.2)	202
Caucasian with epidural	780 (18.7)	4170
Asian, no epidural	52 (15.9)	328
Caucasian, no epidural	614 (10.3)	5965

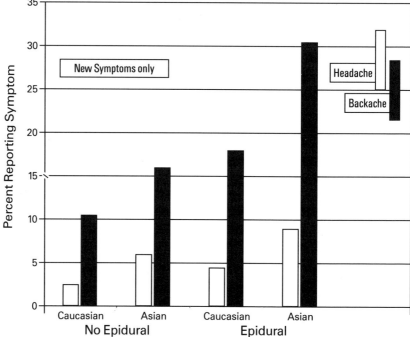

Figure 8.5 Back/Headache, Epidurals, Ethnic Group

TABLE 8.7

Backache, epidural anaesthesia and onset of labour*

	With backache No. (%)	Total
Induced, with epidural	144 (15.3)	941
Spontaneous/augmented, with epidural	700 (20.6)	3399
Induced, no epidural	54 (11.0)	493
Spontaneous/augmented no epidural	639 (10.5)	6098

*Elective sections excluded

TABLE 8.8

Backache, epidural anaesthesia and episiotomy in vaginal deliveries

	Backache No. (%)	Total women
Episiotomy, with epidural	505 (18.8)	2691
Laceration, with epidural	128 (21.1)	608
Intact, with epidural	80 (20.6)	389
Episiotomy, no epidural	257 (10.7)	2405
Laceration, no epidural	230 (10.4)	2221
Intact, no epidural	150 (10.2)	1472

What predicts onsets and durations of backache?

All of the above analyses related to first time backaches, starting within three months of the birth, and persisting longer than six weeks. We did however conduct many additional analyses, including discriminant analyses, for backaches beginning at different times and persisting for different durations. The predominance of epidural anaesthesia as the main predictor of backache remained unaltered throughout.

First we examined different times of onset within and outside the three month limit. Most (82%) of the 1634 backaches that started within three months, began within the first four weeks and many (63%) within the first week. Table 8.9 shows that the epidural association was evident for backaches starting in each of these sub-intervals, but not for onsets beyond the first three months. Newly occurring backaches after this three month limit were **not** associated with epidural anaesthesia.

Table 8.9 also shows the same onset comparisons according to length of second stage labour. Although backache starting in all of the sub-intervals within the first three post-partum months was significantly associated with a long second stage labour, the relationship was strongest for those starting immediately. Like epidural anaesthesia, backache starting more than three months after delivery showed no relationship with a long second stage labour.

Similar forms of analyses were used to examine the associations between epidural anaesthesia and backaches of different durations as opposed to different onset dates. Here the epidural/backache relationship remained constant for backaches of any duration including those which were still persistent at the time of the enquiry (Table 8.10). A long second stage was also associated with backaches of all durations (Table 8.10) but in contrast with the epidural picture it, was more strongly associated with shorter duration backaches than persistent ones. Stated conversely, backaches arising from epidurals seemed more likely to become chronic than backaches arising from long labours.

We also considered onsets and durations of backache in relation to the other predictors such as spinal anaesthesia, and Asian ethnic group, but the numbers were too small for meaningful comparison.

Short-term backache

Although the main scope of this investigation was concerned with longer term health problems after childbirth, we also recorded and analysed symptoms persisting for periods of six weeks or less. Here too there was an association

TABLE 8.9

Differing onsets of backache*, epidural anaesthesia and length of second stage labour

	Onset					
	Within 1 week	2 – 4 weeks	4 weeks – 3 months	3 – 6 months	6 – 12 months	Total women
Epidural	573 (12.02)	172 (3.61)	158 (3.32)	84 (1.76)	67 (1.41)	4766 (100)
No epidural	455 (6.56)	141 (2.03)	135 (1.95)	99 (1.43)	107 (1.54)	6935 (100)
Relative risks	1.83	1.78	1.70	1.23 NS	0.92 NS	
Second Stage						
Up to 1 hour	488 (7.07)	160 (2.32)	157 (2.27)	105 (1.52)	106 (1.54)	6904
1 hour or more	358 (12.97)	98 (3.50)	84 (3.0)	51 (1.82)	44 (1.57)	2798
Relative risks	1.81	1.51	1.32	1.20 NS	0.98 NS	

*For women who had both lower and middle backache, with differing onsets, the earliest onset is given.

TABLE 8.10

Differing durations of backache*, epidural anaesthesia and length of second stage labour

Duration	6 weeks – 3 months No. (%)	3 – 6 months No. (%)	6 – 12 months No. (%)	Over 12 months No. (%)	Still persistent No. (%)	Total Women
Epidural	88 (1.81)	106 (2.22)	83 (1.74)	50 (1.05)	576 (12.1)	4766
No epidural	76 (1.10)	80 (1.15)	52 (0.75)	36 (0.52)	487 (7.0)	6935
Relative risks	1.65	1.93	2.32	2.02	1.73	
Second Stage						
Up to 1 hour	72 (1.04)	83 (1.20)	43 (0.62)	44 (0.64)	563 (8.15)	6904
1 hour or more	67 (2.39)	73 (2.61)	60 (2.14)	27 (0.96)	313 (11.19)	2798
Relative risks	2.30	2.18	3.45	1.50	1.37	

*For women who had both lower and middle backache, with differing durations, the longest duration is given.

between backache and epidural anaesthesia: 2.5% of the women who had an epidural reported newly occurring short-term backache, compared with 1.2% of women with no epidural (RR = 2.08). Short-term backaches are more likely to have been under-reported after such long intervals, so that the recorded frequencies are probably lower than the actual frequencies, but there is no obvious reason why under-reporting should have differed systematically between women who had or did not have epidural anaesthesia.

Discussion

The most striking and specific result to emerge from these data was that women having epidural anaesthesia during labour reported more new and persistent backache than those who did not. The association was statistically 'primary' within the range of available variables, and could not be explained away as an indirect effect. The association was very highly significant and constantly present in a wide range of special situations. An epidural was consistently associated with increased rates of backache in straightforward and in abnormal deliveries: and in many different obstetric circumstances. The relationship did not appear to be an artefact resulting from varied pain tolerance. It was equally evident among backaches of all durations, including those still persisting, and among transient backaches lasting under six weeks. It was equally evident among backaches starting within a week of delivery and for those starting in the second and third months: although not among those starting after three months. The association exhibited the dominance and consistency which one would expect from a cause-effect relationship.

The question then arises what the mechanism of the backache might be; whether it might be an effect of direct needle trauma, or a reaction to the drugs employed, or whether some other explanation might be formulated. The most direct indication of a possible mechanism was found in the data relating to elective Caesarean section. These women experienced no labour and, alone among all the groups, epidural anaesthesia was not associated with any increase in the risk of backache. This suggests that the physical elements of the epidural procedure itself, drug reactions or direct needle trauma, are unlikely to supply the explanation. If that were the case, excess backache should also follow the use of epidural anaesthesia for elective section. Rather it seems that the risk is determined by a combination of sensory and motor loss produced by regional anaesthesia and a period of time in labour; and this is true whether the labour is terminated through vaginal delivery or through emergency section.

The most plausible explanation is that the origin of the backache is postural (MacArthur et al 1990). Stressed postures and uncomfortable positions can occur in any labour. They are sometimes prolonged, without opportunity for movement, especially during the second stage. This itself could cause injury, and later backache could be a direct result. This could arise in non-epidural labours, and we have indeed shown that newly occurring, long-term backache occurred following one in ten deliveries where epidural anaesthesia was **not** used. Under epidural anaesthesia however, there is loss of muscle tone: there is no pain to stimulate movement: and movement in any case generally requires assistance. A women could thus adopt and maintain an 'uncomfortable' and strained position for an extended period. This suggests that the epidural effect is mediated through exacerbating the postural problems of labour: and that the latter are the necessary underlying cause, capable sometimes of generating backache in the absence of anaesthesia.

The independent association observed between backache and a longer second stage further supports the postural hypothesis. That a prolonged second stage seems to have a **greater** effect on backache rates in the absence of an epidural (Table 8.7) suggests that epidural anaesthesia and very prolonged labour to some extent might act as **alternative** mechanisms. Backache induced by long labour seemed generally less persistent than epidural induced backache.

Spinal anaesthesia differs from epidural anaesthesia in that the procedure uses a single-shot technique, followed by withdrawal of the needle. The end-site of the injection also differs in that local anaesthetic is delivered directly into the spinal fluid and no catheter insertion is involved. That backache is also observed following spinal anaesthesia suggests that the common relationship is not mediated through the trauma of an indwelling catheter, and is not dependent upon the specific anatomical location of either injection. However, anaesthetised postural strains remain as a common element of both.

The extremely high rates of backache among Asian women, irrespective of the procedures administered, raise questions which require additional investigation. The Asian women also sought medical advice more often for their backache. Selective reporting biases among different sub-cultures, especially with a postal questionnaire, should be considered alongside other potential causes. However, as we show later the excesses did not follow a pattern consistent with other symptoms, thus suggesting that the higher rates of backache are probably real.

Unlike the durations of the stages of labour, the durations of the epidurals themselves were not recorded within the computerised maternity case records, and we have not yet determined whether the duration, or the dose of the anaesthetic agent, or the stage at which this procedure was administered, affected the risk of subsequent backache. With increasing concentration there is a concomitant increase in the intensity of the motor blockade although some degree can be present with lower concentrations. However these additional data are available from a further set of anaesthetic records, and we shall investigate the effect of alternative durations and concentrations in due course.

Although backaches first occurring between one and three months after delivery, were less common than onsets within the first four weeks, the epidural excess was evident in both groups. This suggests that although the primary 'injury' occurs during delivery, the symptoms are sometimes delayed. Some of these backaches with delayed onsets are doubtless mediated through separate non-childbirth mechanisms, but the continued relationship with the major childbirth predictors suggests that timing must often depend upon an additional precipitating circumstance superimposed upon a latent delivery-injury. We had no data concerning relevant 'lifestyle' variables within these three months, but there are many different activities which could produce back strain during this time, including child-lifting, feeding and extra laundry work. We shall need in the future to pursue the question whether there are any differences in the domestic and employment 'lifestyles' of women who had an epidural, or backache, or both.

We found very little guidance in the medical literature on long term backache first occurring after the delivery of a child. Backache occurring during **pregnancy,** resulting from altered posture, relaxed ligaments and extra weight, and sometimes persisting after delivery, is well documented (e.g. Berg et al, 1988). Short term backache following childbirth has also been reported (Crawford 1972, Grove 1973). However, there was virtually no information relating to newly occurring long term post-partum backache, and particularly in relation to epidural anaesthesia. There is little to indicate that the relationship had even been suspected. For example, a recent textbook on obstetric anaesthesia from the New York Medical Centre (Ramanthan, 1988) includes only a very short note that backache can occur as a consequence of epidural anaesthesia, adding that 'the backache is usually mild and subsides after a few days' (p.102). That is all there is on the matter. Katz et al. (1980) in a paper discussing the complications of spinal and epidural anaesthesia, also note that backache can follow a traumatic needle insertion but they say that it diminishes very quickly. They also comment very briefly that 'a different cause of backache has to do with the muscle relaxation that follows regional anaesthesia. When positioning the patient for various surgical procedures, stretching of ligaments, joint capsules and so on may occur' (p.1220). They do not pursue the issue further.

Kitzinger (1987), reporting on behalf of the National Childbirth Trust, documented the effects of epidural anaesthesia as perceived by women in two self-selected populations. They were replying to questions about epidural anaesthesia and its associated problems, as posed in the National Childbirth Trust magazine and in an Australian Parents' magazine. Self-volunteering respondents are likely to be atypical, and there was no comparison group: the author makes no claims that the findings can be generalised to women at large. Rates relative to non-epidural deliveries could not be calculated, and causal associations could not be proposed; but backache was the most frequently perceived consequence of epidural anaesthesia and is consistent with the results reported here. This information, first published in 1987, was not available to us when we were designing our own investigation.

These few exceptions apart, there appears to be a total lack of published information concerning post-partum backache. The scientific literature contains practically nothing on the magnitude of the problem, or its severity or chronicity, or its highly specfic association with epidural anaesthesia. It is therefore scarcely surprising that the question of a mechanism has never before arisen, and there are no points of cross-reference against which to check our own mechanistic hypothesis. Many different aspects of the epidural backache relationship remain in urgent need of primary investigation before we can begin to unravel the exact details; and thence to formulate possible preventive procedures, and to design preventive or therapeutic trials.

Chapter 9 – Frequent Headaches and Migraine

Headache is a very common complaint which most people experience at times. We therefore restricted our primary question to asking whether the women had experienced **frequent** headaches since having their baby. There was no simple way of defining 'frequent' within a questionnaire administered in this way: the women had to make their own interpretation. We asked a separate question about migraine, again leaving the women to interpret for themselves what migraine was.

Frequency of occurrence

The standard questions on onset, duration, consultation and treatment were repeated for both symptoms. As with other symptoms, the main analysis was based upon frequent headaches or migraine which had begun within three months of the index delivery, had lasted for more than six weeks and had never occurred in this form before. On these criteria, frequent headaches were reported by 419 women (3.6%); and 165 women (1.4%) reported migraine. Among them, 72 women reported both: the total reporting one or the other or both was 512 (4.4%).

An additional 553 (4.7%) women reported frequent post-partum headaches to the same criteria, except that they were not new symptoms; another 662 (5.7%) reported migraine similarly. In contrast with backache, the majority of women with these complaints following the index delivery had also had them previously – 57% for frequent headaches and 80% for migraines. Even among primiparae, 40% and 79% of those with post-partum symptoms had experienced them before this delivery. Clearly, and in contrast with backache, many frequent headaches and migraine were not specifically related to the delivery of a child.

Another 545 women gave inadequately timed reports for their post-partum frequent headaches: and 466 for migraine. Although they had all said that the symptom had occurred following the delivery, they did not date the onset, or give its duration, or say whether or not they had had it before. These reports have been excluded from our analysis. The investigations which follow are limited (unless stated otherwise) to those precisely-dated frequent headaches (419) and migraines (165) which started within three months of the delivery, lasted more than six weeks and had never previously been experienced in that form.

Association between frequent headaches and migraine

The overlaps between responses to the questions on frequent headaches and migraine have been noted. We do not know exactly how many of the 72 women giving double responses wished to indicate two separate problems, and how many had simply indicated the same symptom under two separate headings. However, 47 of the 72 women (60%) reporting both symptoms, declared the onset of each of them in the same post-partum week and reported the same duration. This suggests that most were probably reporting the same symptom twice, under two different heads. Furthermore, although we begin our analyses by studying each symptom separately, we shall show that the statistical associations and symptom predictors of frequent headaches and of migraine are very similar. Later on we consider women with either of these symptoms as an aggregated group.

Durations and onsets

These symptoms were often of long duration. Only 12% of the 419 women with new post-partum headaches said they had lasted for six weeks to three months; the majority (71%) said they had lasted for more than a year: while 63% still had them at the time of questioning. Among those 165 women with new post-partum migraine, only 6% reported cessation within three months; 85% lasted for more than a year; and 76% still had the migraine at the time of the enquiry.

Just over half (53%) of the 419 women first experiencing frequent headaches within three months of delivery, said that they had started within a week; and 74% started within four weeks. For migraine 41% of the 165 women said that this first occurred within the first post-partum week; and 62% within four weeks.

Too long delayed for inclusion in our main analyses, another 152 women reported new long term headaches, beginning between three and twelve months after the birth, making a total of 571 women with long term frequent headaches, starting some time within the first post-partum year. Of this group, 221 (39%) began within the first week; 310 (54%) within the first four weeks and 419 (73%) within the first three months. For migraine a total of 261 women reported first onsets within a year of delivery; with 67 (26%) starting in the first week: 103 (39%) within the first four weeks and 165 (63%) within three months. Although these symptoms are not all childbirth-specific, these timings suggest that some must be precipitated through having a baby.

Medical consultation

Medical consultation rates were greater for frequent headaches and for migraine than for backache; 48% of women with frequent headaches had consulted their doctor, and 60% of those with migraine, compared with 27% for backache. Of those women who reported both headache and migraine, 71% had consulted their doctor. Double reporting might therefore be an indicator of severity.

As with backache, there was no relationship between the rates of medical consultation and the durations of either frequent headaches or migraine: those with long duration symptoms were **not** more likely to consult. Neither were there any social differences (age, ethnic group, etc.) between the women who consulted and those who did not.

Most (76%) of the women with frequent headaches who went to the doctor said they were given treatment. Referral to hospital was uncommon: in only 6% of those attending. Similarly, for migraine, most women who consulted the general practitioner (84%) received treatment, and only 5% were referred for specialist consultation. Those reporting frequent headaches as well as migraine were no more likely to receive treatment or to be referred than those with only one symptom.

Factors associated with frequent headaches and migraine

Table 9.1 and Figure 9.1 illustrate the basic statistical associations of frequent headaches and migraine. The social and demographic associations are set out in the upper part of the table, showing that more symptoms were reported by younger women, unmarried women, those from lower social classes and by Asian women. The Asian excess for migraine was not quite statistically significant at the 5% level. Primiparity was associated with more reports of frequent headache, but not of migraine. These social associations were generally similar to those for backache.

The unstandardised associations with obstetric and anaesthetic factors are given in the lower part of Table 9.1. The picture was less striking than for backache but there were some parallels. Frequent headaches showed a small proportional excess following forceps delivery and emergency Caesarean section. Migraine showed small excesses after forceps delivery and episiotomy. However, as with backache, the greatest enhancement was associated with epidural anaesthesia. This was true both for frequent headaches and for migraine: the separate relative risks were 1.61 and 1.84 respectively, and the joint relative risk for either was 1.59.

TABLE 9.1

Characteristics associated with frequent headaches and with migraine*

Characteristics	Frequent headaches No. (%)	Migraine No. (%)	Total women
Whole sample	419 (3.6)	165 (1.4)	11701
Primiparae	175 (4.2)	52 (1.2) NS	4185
Multiparae	244 (3.2)	113 (1.5)	7516
Under 25 years	155 (5.9)	53 (2.0)	2625
25 – 34	231 (3.0)	97 (1.3)	7688
35 or more	33 (2.4)	15 (1.1)	1388
Married	353 (3.4)	138 (1.3)	10525
Single/Div/Sep/Wid	66 (5.6)	27 (2.3)	1176
Social Class			
I and II	70 (2.4)	24 (0.8)	2882
III, IV & V	247 (3.5)	100 (1.4)	7050
Unemployed	32 (6.1)		525
Caucasian	341 (3.4)	128 (1.3) NS	10135
Asian	39 (7.4)	12 (2.3)	530
Singleton	412 (3.6) NS	157 (1.4)	11532
Multiple	7 (4.1)	8 (4.7)	169
Forceps	101 (4.4)	45 (2.0)	2301
No forceps	318 (3.4)	120 (1.3)	9400
Elective section	25 (3.2)	9 (1.2)	770
Emergency section	56 (4.9)	19 (1.7) NS	1145
Vaginal delivery	338 (3.5)	137 (1.4)	9786
Episiotomy	184 (3.6) NS	87 (1.7)	5112
No episiotomy	235 (3.6)	78 (1.2)	6589
Epidural anaesthesia	220 (4.6)	92 (1.9)	4766
No epidural	199 (4.6)	73 (1.1)	6935

*Symptoms, starting within three months of delivery, never previously experienced and lasting longer than six weeks.

Figure 9.1
Frequent Headaches and Associated Factors

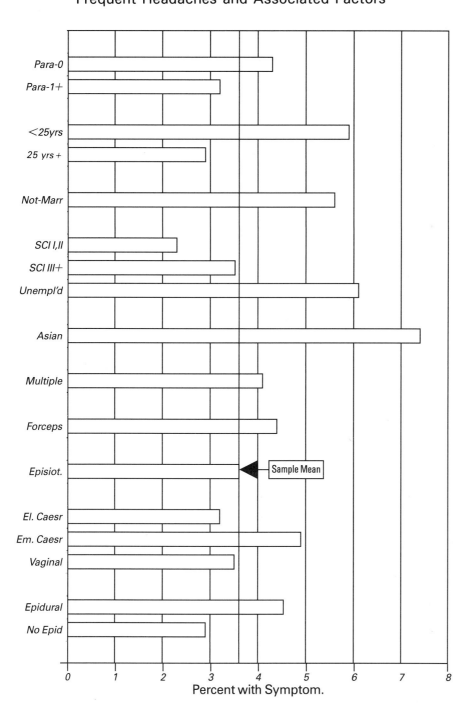

Primary predictors and secondary associations

Discriminant analyses were carried out to determine which of the statistically associated factors predicted each of the symptoms independently, after taking all other factors into account. The standardised associations for frequent headaches are given in Table 9.2, and for migraine in Table 9.3. In each case the analyses were conducted first for vaginal deliveries alone (first two colums), and

TABLE 9.2

Discriminant analysis of characteristics associated with frequent headaches

	Vaginal deliveries		All deliveries	
	F value	Coefficient	F value	Coefficient
Younger age	41.438	0.65239	44.983	0.65980
Epidural	28.688	0.52731	22.158	0.44284
Asian ethnic group	14.149	0.47247	19.374	0.41426
Social class III, IV, V	4.686	0.21930	NS	NS
Emergency section	N/A		4.124	0.19133

TABLE 9.3

Discriminant analysis of characteristics associated with migraine

	Vaginal deliveries		All deliveries	
	F value	Coefficient	F value	Coefficient
Epidural	14.427	0.53481	15.406	0.53496
Multi-parity	13.366	0.55171	14.014	0.53388
Younger age	13.207	0.52762	12.917	0.51080
Twins	10.554	0.42842	12.165	0.45489
Episiotomy	5.0695	0.32871	NS	NS

then for all deliveries together (last two columns). For frequent headaches the predictive social factors were early maternal age, Asian ethnic group and, to a lesser extent, lower social class (III, IV, V). The main obstetric predictor was epidural anaesthesia, with a weaker association for emergency Caesarean section in the second analysis. For migraine the dominant social predictors were multiparity, and earlier maternal age. Multiple pregnancy and episiotomy were also predictive of migraine; but again, the dominant obstetric predictor was epidural anaesthesia.

Social predictors

Parity and age

The problems of interpreting the effects of parity and age have already been encountered and discussed for backache. We generally expect that the limiting criterion of first-time symptoms, will result in bias, with selective inclusion of affected primiparious and younger women. Yet for headache, the discriminant analysis showed **no** independent primiparity excess; and for migraine the association after discriminant analysis was reversed, with symptoms more frequent among multiparae. To examine this further, subsidiary discriminant analysis were conducted, this time for all symptoms starting within three months of delivery and lasting more than six weeks, **irrespective** of whether they were new ones, continuations or recurrences. An association with multiparity then became clearly evident both for frequent headaches and for migraine. To examine the effect of maternal age, additional subsidiary discriminant analyses were conducted for primiparae and multiparae separately, which showed that younger age was a powerful and genuine predictor for both symptoms among both parity groups.

These two predictors, younger age and multiparity, are themselves **inversely** related, so the overall pattern is complex and to some extent paradoxical. In addition primiparity is related to more frequent use of epidural anaesthesia. However the multiparity and the early age relationships were not dispersed by these subsidiary analyses (as had been the case for backache), and they probably reflect real phenomena. We shall return to these points later.

Ethnic group and social class

The excess of frequent headaches among Asian women, compared with Caucasians, remained significant after discriminant analysis, but there was no such association for migraine. This may result from different 'labelling' habits, with Asian women less prone to use the more technical term. The relative risk of headache among Asians was 2.18 compared with Caucasians; a relationship which parallels that found for backache.

Frequent headaches and lower social class remained significantly correlated after discriminant analysis but the social class gradient for migraine disappeared. This might be another labelling effect. Interpretation was again complicated by the selective exclusion of older age groups and higher parities through the 'ever-before?' question, because there were more younger women and more of high parity in the lower social classes (see Chapter 6 and Appendix 2). However, the subsidiary discriminant analysis (above) based upon **all** long term post-delivery headaches, irrespective of past history, failed to disperse the social class association, and indeed enhanced it. Lower social class women might have more social problems relating to income, unemployment and housing, all of which are exacerbated by having a baby. These stressful situations may well give rise to more headaches.

Obstetric and anaesthetic predictors

Epidural anaesthesia

Discriminant analysis confirmed the crude statistical associations between headaches, migraine and epidural anaesthesia and showed that this was the most powerful of the obstetric predictors of both of these symptoms. In this respect the findings resembled those for backache and, as with backache, it was unexpected. We again considered a range of alternative explanations for the relationship.

Epidural anaesthesia, and 'normal deliveries'

The question arises whether the association between headaches and epidural anaesthesia could arise indirectly, because a greater proportion of the epidural deliveries were less straightforward. The discriminant analyses had standardised for the separate indicators of stressful delivery, but had not necessarily excluded the full effects of a composite assessment. We tackled this issue using the technique described for backache. Groups of women with 'normal' and 'abnormal' deliveries (as defined earlier) were examined separately and the results are shown in Table 9.4. This showed on excess of headache (RR = 1.48) due to 'abnormal' delivery in the absence of an epidural (compare rows 2, 4), but not in the presence of an epidural (compare rows 1,3). An epidural showed a major association (RR = 2.04) in 'normal' deliveries (compare rows 1,2), but much less (RR = 1.22) among 'abnormal' deliveries (compare rows 3,4). For migraine the epidural association occurred equally both among 'normal' and 'abnormal' deliveries, with higher symptom rates after an epidural, irrespective of the normality of the delivery. The relationships are expressed graphically in Figure 9.2. There was no evidence here then that

TABLE 9.4

	Frequent headaches No. (%)	Migraine No. (%)	Total women
Frequent headaches, migraine, epidural anaesthesia and 'normal' deliveries			
'Normal' delivery, with epidural	56 (5.1)	20 (1.8)	1098
'Normal' delivery, no epidural	114 (2.5)	45 (1.0)	4646
'Abnormal' delivery, with epidural	164 (4.5)	72 (2.0)	3668
'Abnormal' delivery, no epidural	85 (3.7)	28 (1.2)	2289

Figure 9.2 Headache, Epidurals and 'Normal' Births

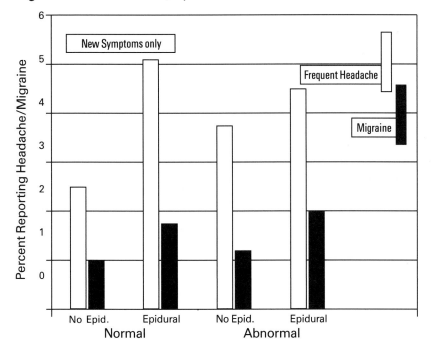

the high rates of frequent headaches or migraine after epidural anaesthesia had arisen indirectly, from the association between epidurals and higher-stress deliveries. Indeed, for frequent headaches there was a degree of **dis**-association between the epidural and the higher stress effects, and they appeared to represent alternative rather than synergistic mechanisms.

Epidural anaesthesia and pain tolerance

As with backache we considered again the question whether variations in pain thresholds might account for associations between epidural anaesthesia and the later complaints of pain. There was no case-note record as to whether the women had themselves requested an epidural for pain relief, or whether they had followed advice to have one: so we identified women with and without a range of medical indications which might precipitate such advice (see Chapter 8). As with backache, we measured the association with an epidural in both groups, also taking account of parity; but no differences between the groups were found (Table 9.5). The result was the same as for backache. There was no evidence that correlated complaints about pain during delivery, and afterwards, could explain the findings.

Epidural anaesthesia and Caesarean section

For backache we had found that an elective Caesarean section differed from other forms of delivery; alone among them, it was not associated with any risk enhancement arising from an epidural. For frequent headaches and for migraine, there was again no risk enhancement from an epidural in women who had an elective section. This time however, there seemed to be no enhancement after emergency section either (Table 9.6). The numbers were small, particularly for migraine, but the epidural association seemed to be limited to vaginal deliveries.

Nevertheless, discriminant analysis showed (Table 9.1, Col. 2) that a Caesarean section, emergency procedures in particular, predicted headache independently of epidural anaesthesia. This was true to the extent that the effect was visible **only** in women who did **not** have an epidural. Table 9.6 shows that there was a significant headache excess after sections without epidural compared with the non-epidural vaginal deliveries. (This difference was statistically significant for emergency sections and in the same direction although non-significant after elective procedures.) This is equivalent to saying that the Caesarean association was limited to women who had general anaesthesia. Here, the neck is extended to facilitate intubation and this may be the source of the problem. We found similar associations for neckache – a phenomenon to be discussed further in Chapter 10.

TABLE 9.5

'Indications' to have epidural and frequent headaches and migraine in vaginal deliveries

	Frequent headaches No. (%)	Migraine No. (%)	Total women
All parities			
Presence of 'indication'	58 (4.37)	27 (2.04)	1326
No 'indication'	119 (5.04)	49 (2.07)	2362
Primiparae			
Presence of 'indication'	32 (5.02)	10 (1.57)	638
No 'indication'	59 (5.0)	21 (1.78)	1178
Multiparae			
Presence of 'indication'	26 (3.78)	17 (2.47)	688
No 'indication'	60 (5.07)	28 (2.36)	1184

TABLE 9.6

Frequent headaches, migraine, type of delivery and epidural anaesthesia

	Frequent headaches No. (%)	Migraine No. (%)	Total women
Vaginal, with epidural	177 (4.8)	76 (2.1)	3688
Vaginal, no epidural	161 (2.6)	61 (1.0)	6098
Emergency section, with epidural	31 (4.8)	10 (1.5)	652
Emergency section, no epidural	25 (5.1)	9 (1.8)	493
Elective section, with epidural	12 (2.8)	6 (1.4)	426
Elective section, no epidural	13 (3.8)	3 (0.9)	344

TABLE 9.7

Frequent headaches, epidural anaesthesia, maternal age and parity

(A) Headache, starting within three months of delivery, duration over six weeks, never had before

Age	Primiparae			
	Epidural		No epidural	
	No. (%)	Total women	No. (%)	Total women
Under 25 years	68 (8.4)	814	27 (3.6)	744
25 – 29 years	32 (3.8)	848	20 (2.9)	679
30 years or more	17 (2.6)	666	10 (2.3)	434

	Multiparae			
	Epidural		No epidural	
	No. (%)	Total women	No. (%)	Total women
Under 25 years	22 (7.5)	292	38 (4.9)	775
25 – 29 years	39 (4.6)	842	57 (3.1)	1856
30 years or more	42 (3.2)	1304	46 (1.9)	2447

(B) Headache, starting within three months of delivery, duration over six weeks irrespective of previous history

Age	Primiparae			
	Epidural		No epidural	
	No. (%)	Total women	No. (%)	Total women
Under 25 years	99 (12.2)	814	67 (9.0)	744
25 – 29 years	59 (7.0)	848	42 (6.2)	679
30 years or more	38 (5.7)	666	27 (6.2)	434

	Multiparae			
	Epidural		No epidural	
	No. (%)	Total women	No. (%)	Total women
Under 25 years	40 (13.7)	292	79 (10.2)	775
25 – 29 years	83 (9.9)	842	155 (8.4)	1856
30 years or more	121 (9.3)	1304	162 (6.6)	2447

TABLE 9.8

Migraine, epidural anaesthesia, maternal age and parity

(A) Migraine, starting within three months of delivery, duration over six weeks, never had before

Age	Primiparae			
	Epidural		No epidural	
	No. (%)	Total women	No. (%)	Total women
Under 25 years	18 (2.2)	814	11 (1.5)	744
25 – 29 years	8 (0.9)	848	1	679
30 years or more	11 (1.7)	666	3 (0.7)	434

Age	Multiparae			
	Epidural		No epidural	
	No. (%)	Total women	No. (%)	Total women
Under 25 years	10 (3.4)	292	14 (1.8)	775
25 – 29 years	18 (2.1)	842	25 (1.3)	1856
30 years or more	27 (2.1)	1304	19 (0.8)	2447

(B) Migraine, starting within three months of delivery, duration over six weeks irrespective of previous history

Age	Primiparae			
	Epidural		No epidural	
	No. (%)	Total women	No. (%)	Total women
Under 25 years	54 (6.6)	814	47 (6.3)	74
25 – 29 years	50 (5.9)	848	31 (4.6)	679
30 years or more	50 (7.5)	666	17 (3.9)	434

Age	Multiparae			
	Epidural		No epidural	
	No. (%)	Total women	No. (%)	Total women
Under 25 years	30 (10.3)	292	56 (7.2)	775
25 – 29 years	70 (8.3)	842	154 (8.3)	1856
30 years or more	110 (8.4)	1304	158 (6.5)	2447

Epidural anaesthesia, parity and age

The complexity of the relationships between headache and migraine and parity, maternal age, and epidural anaesthesia, led us to examine combination of these factors in more detail, as shown in Tables 9.7 and 9.8. Women with first time symptoms are tabulated in Panel A; and all post-partum complaints, first-time or not, are tabulated in Panel B. The negative age-gradient for frequent headaches occurred everywhere in Table 9.7, with the highest rates in women under twenty-five years of age. This withstood all attempts to explain it in terms of the biased exclusions of women who had had the symptoms before (Panel B). The effect of increasing parity was also consistently present in all cells where comparison was possible. The effect of epidural anaesthesia also remained constant, clearly visible in every cell of the table where the numbers were sufficient. Table 9.8 shows the same analysis for migraine: the numbers were too small here to permit such definite conclusions but the age, parity and epidural relationships were similar.

Epidural anaesthesia and ethnic group

Detailed cross-tabulations of ethnic group and epidural anaesthesia are shown in Table 9.9. This re-confirmed that the epidural effect was independent of ethnic group; and it showed very high rates of headache in Asian women, irrespective of whether they had epidural anaesthesia. These findings resemble those for backache. For migraine neither the crude nor the multivariate Asian

TABLE 9.9

Frequent headaches, epidural anaesthesia and Asian ethnic group		
	Frequent headaches	Total women
	No. (%)	
Asian, with epidural	19 (9.4)	202
Caucasian, with epidural	201 (4.4)	4170
Asian, no epidural	20 (6.1)	328
Caucasian, no epidural	179 (2.6)	5965

excess was quite statistically significant, although the gradients were in the same direction. The numbers were too small for three-way cross tabulation.

Other obstetric predictors

Two additional obstetric predictors of migraine are shown in Table 9.3: multiple pregnancy and episiotomy. For multiple pregnancy the numbers were small: only 8 cases of migraine in twins compared with two cases expected; and the association with episiotomy was only a weak one.

Spinal headache

A spinal headache was recorded in the maternity case-notes as a 'complication of the puerperium' in 34 women. This refers to the characteristic postural headache following either 'spinal' anaesthesia (13) or an accidental dural puncture during epidural anaesthesia (21). This type of headache is generally considered to subside, even if untreated, within about a week (Brownridge 1983). However among these 34 women the headache was reported to be long lasting by nine women (25%). Five of these long-term headaches followed a dural tap (0.1% of all epidurals administered) and four were after a spinal block (2.5% of all spinals administered). Kitzinger (1987) in her descriptive study of epidurals (see Chapter 8) noted that among twelve women who had dural taps, some (no number given) had headaches which persisted for many weeks.

Short-term headaches

The above results all relate to symptoms lasting more than six weeks, but we also examined relationships between epidural anaesthesia and headaches lasting for six weeks or less. This examination yielded a similar picture. Among the 83 women who reported new short-term headaches, there was a significant excess (RR = 2.0) after an epidural.

Inter-relationships between backache, headache and migraine

There were close relationships between the occurrence of headache, migraine and backache. Among the women reporting headache, 160 (38%) also reported backache; and of those reporting migraine, 61 (37%) also reported backache.

This is 3.9 times the frequency of backache in women without headache or migraine. Frequent headaches and migraine showed similar associations and common predictors and these same factors also predicted backache. We therefore examined combinations of these symptoms in more detail, using discriminant analyses to identify the most powerful predictors of each symptom alone, and in combination with the others. These analyses showed that for backache alone, and for backache combined with either headache or migraine, epidural anaesthesia remained the dominant predictor. But where either headache or migraine were experienced alone, it was not. The main predictive factors in these last cases were early maternal age and multiparity. Asian ethnic group was also an important predictor of backache alone and of headache combined with backache, but not of headache in the absence of backache.

The relationships between these three symptoms and their combinations were simultaneously cross-tabulated against epidural anaesthesia, confirming the results of the discriminant analyses. This examination also revealed that headache with backache seemed even more closely related to epidural anaesthesia than was backache alone (Table 9.10). The cross-tabulation shown in Table 9.11 also confirmed the predictive power of primiparity and advancing maternal age. The highest rates of headache/migraine without backache occurred among women aged under 25 years with more than one child, irrespective of epidural anaesthesia.

TABLE 9.10

Headache, migraine and backache and epidural anaesthesia

Combinations of all three symptoms

	Epidural No. (%)	No epidural No. (%)	RR
Headache alone	98 (2.06)	123 (1.77)	1.16
Migraine alone	30 (0.63)	36 (0.52)	1.21
Backache alone	783 (16.4)	664 (9.60)	1.72
Headache + migraine	19 (0.40)	19 (0.27)	1.48
Headache + backache	77 (1.62)	49 (0.71)	2.28
Migraine + backache	17 (0.36)	10 (0.14)	2.57
Headache, migraine + backache	26 (0.55)	8 (0.12)	4.58
None of these 3 symptoms	3716 (78.0)	6026 (86.9)	0.90
Totals	4766 (100)	6935 (100)	

TABLE 9.11

Headache, migraine and backache, epidural anaesthesia, parity and age

Primiparae

| | Epidural | | | No Epidural | | |
Age	Just head/ migraine No. (%)	Head/mig/ + back No. (%)	Total women	Just head/ migraine No. (%)	Head/mig/ + back No. (%)	Total women
Under 25 years	30 (3.7)	46 (5.7)	814	20 (2.7)	12 (1.6)	744
25 yrs or more	34 (2.2)	26 (1.7)	1514	20 (1.8)	14 (1.3)	1113
All ages	64 (2.7)	72 (3.1)	2328	40 (2.2)	26 (1.4)	1857

Multiparae

| | Epidural | | | No Epidural | | |
Age	Just head/ migraine No. (%)	Head/mig/ + back No. (%)	Total women	Just head/ migraine No. (%)	Head/mig/ + back No. (%)	Total women
Under 25 years	18 (6.2)	10 (3.4)	292	40 (5.2)	8 (1.0)	775
25 yrs or more	65 (3.0)	38 (1.8)	2146	98 (2.3)	33 (0.8)	4303
All ages	83 (3.4)	48 (2.0)	2438	138 (2.7)	41 (0.8)	5078

What predicts onsets and duration of frequent headaches and migraine?

As with backache, we analysed detailed times of onsets within the defining three months post-partum period, and for onsets after this. We also repeated these analyses for different durations, beyond six weeks. None of these examinations caused us to question the picture of symptom predictors so far described.

Onset dates for women who had headache/migraine alone, for those with backache alone, and for those with the combined symptoms are shown in Panel A of Table 9.12. The onsets for headache alone were more evenly spread than for the other two, although almost half started within a week of delivery. Panel B cross-tabulates onsets of combined symptoms according to whether or not they

TABLE 9.12

Differing onsets of symptoms in women with headache alone, backache alone and combined symptoms

(A)	Onset within 1 week No. (%)	2 – 4 weeks No. (%)	5 – 13 weeks No. (%)	Total women
Headache alone	146 (44.9)	73 (22.5)	106 (32.6)	325
Backache alone	913 (63.1)	274 (18.9)	260 (18.0)	1447
Headache + backache				
Headache onset	115 (61.5)	37 (19.8)	35 (18.7)	187
Backache onset	127 (68.0)	30 (16.0)	30 (16.0)	187

(B) Combined symptoms and epidural anaesthesia

	Onset within 1 week No. (%)	2 – 4 weeks No. (%)	5 – 13 weeks No. (%)	Total women
Headache onset after epidural	85 (70.8)	17 (14.2)	18 (15.0)	120
Headache onset, no epidural	30 (44.8)	20 (29.9)	17 (25.4)	67
Backache onset after epidural	86 (71.7)	17 (14.2)	17 (14.2)	120
Backache onset, no epidural	41 (61.2)	13 (19.4)	13 (19.4)	67

followed epidural anaesthesia. It shows that those symptoms which followed an epidural were much more likely to be immediate (71%). In fact among the 120 women with combined headache and backache following epidural, 67 (56%) reported both symptoms as immediate: 18 said headache started immediately, backache later; and 19 reported the reverse. This makes a total of 104 (87%) out of the 120 shown in the Table where one or both symptoms had started immediately; and a second-week onset was reported in a further nine cases. The clustering around delivery in this group was striking.

Headaches starting within the first post-partum year but after the first three months were unrelated to epidural anaesthesia: the same pattern as for backache. However headaches beginning any time during the first year continued to be associated with multiparity: but only where they occurred alone and not combined with backache (Table 9.13).

We made similar comparisons of the symptoms and their combinations according to their differing durations, but found nothing of note. All durations were equally represented among headaches occurring alone and those combined with backache; and following or not following an epidural; and in older women with more than one child.

TABLE 9.13

Differing onsets of headache/migraine with and without backache and parity

	Onset within 1 week No. (%)	2 – 4 weeks No. (%)	5 – 13 weeks No. (%)	3 – 12 months No. (%)	Total women
(A) Headache/migraine without backache					
Primiparae	43 (1.03)	22 (0.53)	39 (0.93)	52 (1.24)	4185
Multiparae	103 (1.37)	51 (0.68)	67 (0.89)	117 (1.56)	7516
Relative risks	1.33	1.28	0.96	1.26	
(B) Headache/migraine with backache					
Primiparae	64 (1.53)	19 (0.45)	15 (0.36)	24 (0.57)	4185
Multiparae	51 (0.68)	20 (0.27)	18 (0.24)	18 (0.24)	7516
Relative risks	0.44	0.60	0.67	0.42	

Discussion

Two published investigations have shown that between 30% and 40% of women experienced a headache on at least one day among the seven days following delivery (Pitt 1973; Stein et al. 1984;). An association between these headaches and previous migraine was also demonstrated (Stein 1981). It has been shown that a small proportion of women experience dural tap during epidural anaesthesia, which can result in severe headaches lasting up to several days after the birth (Crawford 1972). However, we have not found any previous investigation of headaches persisting beyond the immediate post-partum period. Once more, the literature is empty.

Our own results indicate that long term frequent headaches, and/or migraine, newly occurring within three months of delivery, were reported by one in 20 women (4.4%). The patterns of associations and the identified predictors were so similar for these two complaints that they can be regarded as interchangeable terms in this context. For this reason we subsequently analysed them as an aggregated group. The only exception to their apprarent equivalence was in relation to ethnic group: in contrast with headaches, migraine showed no excess among Asian women, although this could be a question of language and labelling differences.

To our surprise we found that epidural anaesthesia was strongly associated with new post partum frequent headaches and migraine, and there was a broad pattern of correlations which bore a strong resemblance to those already encountered with backache. There was also a strong correlation between occurrences of headache/migraine and backache. Like backache, there was no evidence that the association between an epidural and headache/migraine resulted from an excess of 'abnormal' deliveries among women having the procedure, or from an excessive reaction to pain in women accepting or requesting it.

We found that when the frequent headaches or migraine were unaccompanied by backache then associations differed from those of headache combined with backache. These combined symptoms showed no parity-association and only a weak maternal age association: but was closely associated with epidural anaesthesia. The epidural-related headaches and backaches displayed a striking degree of clustering around delivery, with 84% starting within the first post-partum week. By contrast, headache/migraine without backache occurred more often in young, multiparous women, and was only marginally related to epidural anaesthesia. These unaccompanied headaches began at any time within the three month post partum period: and indeed after this time, throughout the whole of the first year. This suggests that headache on its own is probably related primarily to continuing social and environmental pressures upon younger mothers caring for more than one child: we would not expect such effects to cluster as closely around the time of birth as the combined symptoms, with their clear relationships with delivery factors.

The high frequency of reported headaches among Asian women was similar to the finding for backache. This excess was only for headache accompanied by backache, not headache alone. This pattern might have resulted from cultural variations in the description of pain or of reaction to pain, or in the willingness to report it. However, if cultural reporting bias provided the whole explanation we would have expected similar ethnic differences among those reporting headache alone. The Asian excess of headache with backache was also strongly related to epidural anaesthesia. This suggests that the ethnic differences could be genuine, and that they merit further investigation.

These findings support the hypothesis that there are two distinct 'syndromes' of post-partum headache/migraine. The first is usually combined with backache, is associated with epidural anaesthesia, has an early and often immediate onset, and is frequent among Asian women. We postulate that this forms part of a wider spinal-axis 'syndrome' with postural origins, dominated by backache, with headache as one of its less frequent symptoms. The second 'syndrome' consists of headache unaccompanied by backache and is associated with the environmental stresses of child care under difficult circumstances; it is neither postural nor associated with epidurals, and it occurs more frequently among younger, multiparous women.

Chapter 10 – Additional Musculo-Skeletal Symptoms

The analyses presented in the last two chapters identified a group of post-partum backaches, sometimes accompanied by frequent headaches or migraine, whose risk was exacerbated by epidural anaesthesia. We hypothesised that the common explanation was a posturally-determined injury, and we formulated the idea of a 'spinal axis syndrome' of which both symptoms were a part. Other women had frequent headaches or migraine without accompanying backache but their symptoms were not related to epidural anaesthesia, were determined mainly through social pressures, and amounted to a separate 'syndrome'.

Several other musculo-skeletal symptoms recorded on the questionnaire could have been secondary to these postural injuries, and might appear as additional extensions of the 'spinal axis syndrome'. In this chapter we therefore examine their relationship with backache and headache and their relationship with epidural anaesthesia – as well as a number of other obstetric and social factors. These symptoms include neckache; shoulderache; pain in the arms and in the legs; weakness in the arms and in the legs; and tingling in the arms and in the legs. All eight were individually infrequent, compared with backache or headache/migraine, although 8.2% of the women complained of at least one of them.

Frequency of occurrence

The proportions of women reporting these musculo-skeletal symptoms ranged from 0.9% (108) for pain in the arms, to 2.5% (293) for tingling in the hands and fingers (Table 10.1, Column 1). These proportions relate to the standard definitions – new symptoms beginning within three months of the index delivery, and lasting longer than six weeks. The second column of Table 10.1 includes recurrences or continuations of symptoms previously experienced. The third column shows the proportions of primiparae for whom the symptoms were first-time occurrences, giving an indication of the degree of childbirth-specificity. These proportions, ranging between 61% and 74%, were similar to the 72% noted for backache, and much greater than the less specific 40% and 21% for frequent headaches and migraine.

The final column of Table 10.1 gives the numbers of additional women who reported inadequately dated symptoms: they supplied no information on the onset, or on the duration, or else did not say whether the symptom was a new one. As with backache, this suggests that the above estimates of prevalence must be higher. These groups were nevertheless excluded from our main analyses so that our findings would be based on firm data, related specifically to the index delivery.

TABLE 10.1

Frequencies of symptoms

	Occurred within 3 mths: Over 6 weeks: First time	Occurred within 3 mths: Over 6 weeks	First time symptoms among primiparae	Additional reports excluded with inadequate dating
	No. (%)	No. (%)	%	No.
Neckache	228 (1.9)	410 (3.5)	63	204
Shoulderache	263 (2.2)	471 (4.0)	61	204
Pain in arms	108 (0.9)	186 (1.6)	66	88
Pain in legs	240 (2.1)	509 (4.4)	62	187
Weak arms	142 (1.2)	210 (1.8)	74	107
Weak legs	148 (1.3)	248 (2.1)	67	77
Tingling hands	293 (2.5)	538 (4.6)	64	290
Tingling feet	126 (1.1)	226 (1.9)	66	81

Durations and onsets

All the included symptoms had lasted for at least six weeks, but most lasted much longer. The distributions of the different durations are shown in Table 10.2. Only a few lasted three months or less, the proportion ranging from 8% for pain in the arms to 15% for shoulderache. Most lasted more than a year, ranging from 66% for weakness in the arms, to 76% for pains in the arms. Many had not subsided at the time of enquiry, thirteen months to nine years later. Unresolved symptoms ranged from 58% for weakness in the legs, to 68% for neckache. This tendency towards chronicity resembled that already noted for backache and for headache.

All onsets up to three months were included in the main analyses, but many symptoms had started within a week. These proportions (Table 10.3, Column 2) ranged from 44% for pain in the arms, to 63% for weakness in the legs.

Table 10.3 also gives numbers of new long term symptoms beginning throughout the whole of the first year (Column 3), and the proportions of these which began in the first week (Column 4), and in the first three months (Column

TABLE 10.2

Duration of musculo-skeletal symptoms

	1	2	3	4
	Total number reported symptoms	Prop. (of 1) lasting up to 3 months	Prop. (of 1) lasting over one year	Prop. (of 1) with persistent symptoms
Neckache	228	12%	72%	68%
Shoulderache	263	15%	67%	59%
Pain in arms	108	8%	76%	65%
Pain in legs	240	12%	68%	60%
Weak arms	142	15%	66%	61%
Weak legs	148	13%	66%	58%
Tingling hands	293	11%	72%	66%
Tingling feet	126	11%	71%	62%
Backache	1634	10%	70%	65%
Headaches	512	9%	76%	68%

TABLE 10.3

Onsets of musculo-skeletal symptoms

	1		2		
	Total No. reporting symptoms in 3 mths*	Prop. (of 1) starting in first week	Total No. reporting symptoms in 12 mths*	Prop. (of 2) starting in first week	Prop. (of 2) starting within 3 mths
Neckache	228	54%	327	38%	70%
Shoulderache	263	50%	368	36%	71%
Pain in arms	108	44%	164	29%	66%
Pain in legs	240	59%	334	42%	72%
Weak arms	142	56%	186	43%	76%
Weak legs	148	63%	193	48%	77%
Tingling hands	293	54%	424	37%	69%
Tingling feet	126	58%	168	43%	75%
Backache	1634	63%	1991	52%	82%
Headaches	512	51%	723	36%	71%

*In all cases these numbers include only symptoms that had persisted for more than six weeks and which were first time occurrences since the index delivery.

5). First week onsets ranged from 29% to 48% and first-quarter onsets from 66% to 77%. Those starting after three months were not included in the main analyses. These proportions of early onsets provide an additional indicator of the childbirth-specificity of the different symptoms.

Pain in the arms was the least childbirth-specific of the musculo-skeletal symptoms, although 66% occurred in the first three months of the year. At the other extreme, 48% of first-year occurrences of weakness in the legs had commenced within a week of delivery, and 77% within three months. These timings suggest a childbirth connection for many of the symptoms.

Medical consultation

For each symptom we asked whether the woman had consulted a doctor. Consultation rates for these musculo-skeletal symptoms were substantially greater than for backache, and comparable with headache; they ranged from 36% for shoulderache to 53% for pain in the legs and 56% for pain in the arms (Table 10.4, Column 1). For backache we had recorded only 27%: for frequent headaches, 48%.

TABLE 10.4

Medical consultation, treatment and referral of musculo-skeletal symptoms

	1 Consulted a Doctor		2 Given treat-ment without referral		3 Referral	
	No.	% of total with symptom	No.	(% of 1)	No.	(% of 1)
Neckache	92	(40)	54	(59)	19	(21)
Shoulderache	95	(36)	56	(59)	17	(18)
Pain in arms	61	(56)	33	(54)	16	(26)
Pain in legs	126	(53)	58	(46)	20	(16)
Weak arms	67	(47)	27	(40)	21	(31)
Weak legs	55	(37)	25	(45)	14	(25)
Tingling hands	113	(39)	33	(29)	35	(31)
Tingling feet	57	(45)	14	(25)	17	(30)
Backache	488	(30)	298	(61)	65	(13)
Headaches	201	(48)	153	(76)	13	(6)

TABLE 10.5

Characteristics associated with musculo-skeletal symptoms*

	Neckache No. (%)	Shoulder-ache No. (%)	Pain in arms No. (%)	Pain in legs No. (%)	Weakness in arms No. (%)	Weakness in legs No. (%)	Tingling in hands/ fingers No. (%)	Tingling in feet/ toes No. (%)	Total women
Whole sample	228 (1.9)	263 (2.2)	108 (0.9)	240 (2.1)	142 (1.2)	148 (1.3)	293 (2.5)	126 (1.1)	11701
Primiparae	105 (2.5)	119 (2.8)	41 (1.0) NS	94 (2.2) NS	50 (1.2) NS	58 (1.4) NS	109 (2.6) NS	53 (1.3) NS	4185
Multiparae	123 (1.6)	144 (1.9)	67 (0.9)	146 (1.9)	92 (1.2)	90 (1.2)	184 (2.4)	73 (1.0)	7516
Under 25 years	60 (2.3)	60 (2.3)	25 (1.0)	82 (3.1)	28 (1.1)	40 (1.5)	64 (2.4)	32 (1.2)	2625
25 – 29 years	90 (2.1) NS	102 (2.4) NS	31 (0.7) NS	60 (1.4)	44 (1.0) NS	55 (1.3) NS	103 (2.4) NS	45 (1.1) NS	4225
30 or more	78 (1.6)	101 (2.1)	52 (1.1)	90 (2.0)	70 (1.4)	53 (1.1)	126 (2.6)	49 (1.0)	4851
Married	202 (1.9) NS	236 (2.2) NS	95 (0.9) NS	212 (2.0) NS	126 (1.2) NS	122 (1.2) NS	258 (2.5) NS	110 (1.0) NS	10525
Single/Div/Wid/Sep	26 (2.2)	27 (2.3)	13 (1.1)	28 (2.4)	16 (1.4)	26 (2.2)	35 (3.0)	16 (1.4)	1176
Caucasian	189 (1.9) NS	225 (2.2)	78 (0.8)	178 (1.8)	103 (1.0)	111 (1.1)	247 (2.4) NS	101 (1.0) NS	10135
Asian	14 (2.6)	19 (3.6)	19 (3.6)	34 (6.4)	25 (4.7)	24 (4.5)	20 (3.8)	9 (1.7)	503
Height under 155cms	22 (1.5)	30 (2.1)	23 (1.6)	37 (2.6)	26 (1.8)	19 (1.3)	43 (3.0)	16 (1.1)	1435
155 – 164cms	140 (2.3) NS	160 (2.6) NS	53 (0.9)	112 (1.9) NS	68 (1.1)	79 (1.3) NS	170 (2.8)	74 (1.2) NS	6037
165 cms or more	54 (1.5)	61 (1.8)	26 (0.8)	68 (2.0)	38 (1.1)	34 (1.0)	69 (2.0)	29 (0.8)	3466
Hypertension	23 (2.2) NS	16 (1.5) NS	7 (0.7) NS	20 (1.9) NS	10 (0.9) NS	13 (1.2) NS	34 (3.2)	15 (1.4) NS	1055
No hypertension	205 (1.9)	247 (2.3)	101 (0.9)	220 (2.1)	132 (1.2)	135 (1.3)	259 (2.4)	111 (1.0)	10646
1st stage labour									
Under 2 hours	26 (1.3)	34 (1.7)	14 (0.7)	29 (1.4)	25 (1.2)	19 (0.9)	36 (1.8)	13 (0.6)	2054
2 – 5 hrs 59 mins	94 (1.8)	97 (1.8)	44 (0.8) NS	95 (1.8)	62 (1.2) NS	54 (1.0)	136 (2.6)	47 (0.9)	5264
6 hours or more	56 (2.6)	64 (2.9)	20 (0.9)	69 (3.1)	29 (1.3)	39 (1.8)	65 (3.0)	32 (1.5)	2195
2nd stage labour									
Up to 15 mins	46 (1.5)	45 (1.5)	22 (0.7)	52 (1.7)	35 (1.2)	31 (1.0)	63 (2.1)	27 (0.9)	3014
16 – 59 mins	64 (1.6)	84 (2.2)	32 (0.8) NS	79 (2.0)	42 (1.1)	45 (1.2) NS	92 (2.4)	38 (1.0)	3891
60 – 119 mins	47 (2.5)	46 (2.5)	13 (0.7)	34 (1.8)	23 (1.2)	26 (1.4)	53 (2.9)	11 (0.6)	1858
120 mins or more	22 (2.3)	25 (2.7)	13 (1.4)	30 (3.2)	19 (2.0)	15 (1.6)	31 (3.3)	18 (1.9)	929

TABLE 10.5 Cont.

	Neckache No. (%)	Shoulder-ache No. (%)	Pain in arms No. (%)	Pain in legs No. (%)	Weakness in arms No. (%)	Weakness in legs No. (%)	Tingling in hands/ fingers No. (%)	Tingling in feet/ toes No. (%)	Total women
Forceps	54 (2.3) NS	57 (2.5) NS	18 (0.8) NS	54 (2.3) NS	39 (1.7)	36 (1.6) NS	68 (3.0) NS	33 (1.4) NS	2301
No forceps	174 (1.9)	206 (2.2)	90 (1.0)	186 (2.0)	103 (1.1)	112 (1.2)	225 (2.4)	93 (1.0)	9400
Caesarean section	50 (2.6)	64 (3.3)	30 (1.6)	45 (2.3) NS	24 (1.3) NS	31 (1.6) NS	53 (2.8) NS	34 (1.8)	1915
Vaginal delivery	178 (1.8)	199 (2.0)	78 (0.8)	195 (2.0)	118 (1.2)	117 (1.2)	240 (2.5)	92 (0.9)	9786
PPH	32 (2.2) NS	16 (1.5) NS	22 (1.5)	29 (2.0) NS	19 (1.3) NS	24 (1.6) NS	46 (3.1) NS	26 (1.7)	1487
No PPH	196 (1.9)	247 (2.3)	86 (0.8)	211 (2.1)	123 (1.2)	124 (1.2)	247 (2.4)	100 (1.0)	10214
Epidural	116 (2.4)	126 (2.6)	54 (1.1)	102 (2.1) NS	65 (1.4) NS	61 (1.3) NS	143 (3.0)	64 (1.3)	4766
No epidural	112 (1.6)	137 (2.0)	54 (0.8)	138 (2.0)	77 (1.1)	87 (1.3)	150 (2.2)	62 (0.9)	6935
Pethidine	38 (2.3) NS	43 (2.6) NS	15 (0.9) NS	41 (2.5) NS	28 (1.7) NS	30 (1.8)	55 (3.3)	18 (1.1) NS	1658
No pethidine	190 (1.9)	220 (2.2)	93 (0.9)	199 (2.0)	114 (1.1)	118 (1.2)	238 (2.4)	108 (1.1)	10043
Tranquilliser	12 (1.8) NS	16 (2.4) NS	7 (1.0) NS	23 (3.4)	8 (1.2) NS	6 (0.9) NS	17 (2.5) NS	5 (0.7) NS	673
No tranquilliser	216 (2.0)	247 (2.2)	101 (0.9)	217 (2.0)	134 (1.2)	142 (1.3)	276 (2.5)	121 (1.1)	1028
General anaesthesia	33 (2.8)	41 (3.5)	16 (1.4) NS	29 (2.5) NS	17 (1.5) NS	24 (2.1)	29 (2.5) NS	17 (1.5) NS	1158
No GA	195 (2.8)	222 (2.1)	92 (0.9)	211 (2.0)	125 (1.2)	124 (1.2)	264 (2.5)	109 (1.0)	10543
Birthweight									
Up to 3200 grams	81 (1.8)	104 (2.4)	46 (1.1)	97 (2.2)	58 (1.3)	63 (1.4)	97 (2.2)	49 (1.1)	4380
3201 – 3700 grams	96 (2.1) NS	104 (2.3) NS	35 (0.8) NS	87 (1.9) NS	56 (1.2) NS	56 (1.2) NS	110 (2.4)	39 (0.9) NS	4557
3701 grams or more	51 (1.8)	55 (2.0)	27 (1.0)	56 (2.0)	28 (1.0)	29 (1.0)	86 (3.1)	38 (1.4)	2764
Head circumference									
Up to 32 cms	31 (2.4)	29 (2.2)	20 (1.5)	37 (2.8)	16 (1.2)	25 (1.9)	28 (2.1)	16 (1.2)	1317
33 – 34 cms	89 (1.8) NS	117 (2.4) NS	43 (0.9)	99 (2.0) NS	68 (1.4) NS	57 (1.2)	127 (2.6) NS	56 (1.1) NS	4904
35 cms or more	107 (2.0)	116 (2.1)	45 (0.8)	102 (1.9)	58 (1.1)	65 (1.2)	138 (2.6)	54 (1.0)	5408

*Musculo-skeletal symptoms starting within three months of delivery, never previously experienced, lasting longer than six weeks

The proportions of those consulting who then received treatment are shown in Column 2. They varied considerably from 25% of those consulting with tingling in the feet or toes, to 59% for neckache and shoulderache; but all were lower than for backache and headache. On the other hand, referral rates among those who consulted were higher than for backache and much higher than for headache. They ranged from 16% for pain in the legs, to 31% for tingling in the hands or fingers. Clearly, many of the symptoms were not regarded by their doctors as trivial complaints.

Factors associated with musculo-skeletal symptoms

As with backache and headache, we first examined the simple statistical associations between musculo-skeletal symptoms and the social and demographic characteristics of the mothers. They are shown in the top part of Table 10.5 and in Figures 10.1 and 10.2. There was more neckache and more shoulderache in primiparae. Early maternal age was associated with pain in the legs; unmarried women reported more weakness in the legs; and shorter women had more weakness and pain in the arms and tingling in the hands. However, the dominant social factor associated with many of these symptoms was ethnic group: Asian women were much more likely to report almost all of them. Only for neckache and tingling in the hands and feet were the differences not statistically significant, although they were still in the same direction. There were only 530 Asian women in the sample, so the numbers affected were small, but the relative risks were high. For pains and weakness in the arms and legs the relative risks in Asian women, compared with Caucasian women, were between 3.5 and 4.5.

The obstetric and anaesthetic associations of the musculo skeletal symptoms are given in the lower part of Table 10.5. None of the antenatal factors were correlated, but the durations of the first and second stages of labour were associated with most of these symptoms. Forceps delivery was associated only with weakness in the arms. Caesarean section was associated with higher rates of several symptoms: neckache, shoulderache, pain in the arms, and tingling in the feet. Post-partum haemorrhage, itself statistically related to Caesarean section, was also significantly associated with the last two symptoms. Epidural and general anaesthesia were associated with several symptoms; pethidine and tranquillisers with only a few; spinal and pudendal block with none. Increased birthweight was associated with tingling in the hands, and greater head circumference with pain in the arms and weakness in the legs.

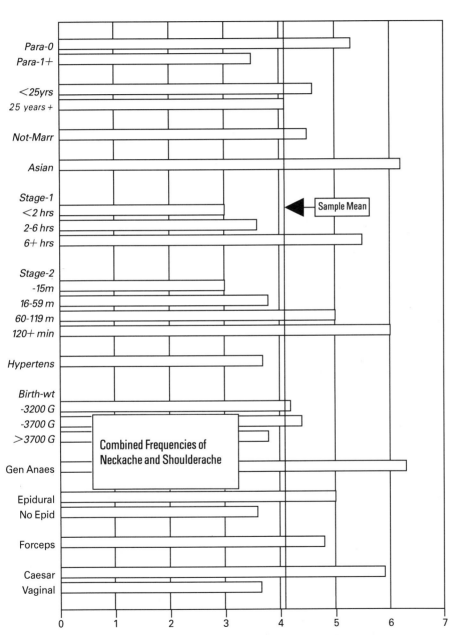

Figure 10.1

Neck/Shoulder Ache & Associated Factors

Para-0
Para-1+

<25yrs
25 years +

Not-Marr

Asian

Stage-1
<2 hrs
2-6 hrs
6+ hrs

Stage-2
-15m
16-59 m
60-119 m
120+ min

Hypertens

Birth-wt
-3200 G
-3700 G
>3700 G

Gen Anaes

Epidural
No Epid

Forceps

Caesar
Vaginal

Sample Mean

Combined Frequencies of
Neckache and Shoulderache

Symptoms/100 Women.

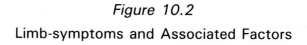

Figure 10.2
Limb-symptoms and Associated Factors

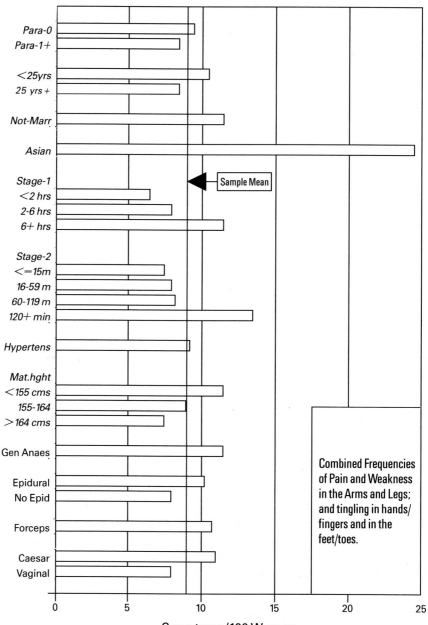

Symptoms/100 Women.

Primary predictors and secondary associations

Many of the associated factors were themselves inter-related, and likely to generate a range of secondary statistical associations. Discriminant analyses were therefore conducted to identify the primary predictors. In keeping with earlier practice, two analyses were carried out for each symptom, the first for vaginal deliveries only, incorporating durations of the stages of labour as variables; the second for all deliveries, with Caesarean section included as a variable, but no duration of labour. The results are in Table 10.6.

Social predictors

Under discriminant analysis, several social, obstetric and anaesthetic factors predicted different musculo-skeletal symptoms, and some predicted more than one (Table 10.6). Comprehensive cross-tabulations, as used in previous chapters, were less practical because of the smaller numbers of affected women but a limited analysis was undertaken and a number of pertinent points emerged, as described below.

Ethnic group

The main social predictor of musculo-skeletal symptoms was Asian ethnic group. For pain in the arms and in the legs, and for weakness in the arms and in the legs, this was the dominant risk-discriminator among all social, obstetric, and anaesthetic factors. It was also a significant predictor for shoulder ache, although to a lesser extent.

Asian ethnic group was shown earlier to be a highly significant predictor of backache and of frequent headaches, especially where these occurred together. We therefore examined all the musculo-skeletal symptoms as a group, including headache and backache, in order to clarify the overall pattern of symptoms among the Asian women. First we counted the total number of musculo-skeletal symptoms (including backaches and headaches) among the 530 Asian women. There were 355: a mean of 0.67 symptoms per woman. Among the 10135 Caucasian women 3251 musculo-skeletal symptoms were reported, a mean of 0.32 per woman; only half as many as the Asian women. The differences were most striking for pains and weakness in the arms and legs; there were 102 reports of these among the Asian women, a mean of 0.2; compared with 470 among the Caucasian women and a mean of 0.05. This represents a fourfold Asian excess.

We looked for clustering of musculo-skeletal symptoms among the Asians to see whether a few women perhaps accounted for most of the symptom reports,

TABLE 10.6

Discriminant analyses of musculo-skeletal symptoms

	Vaginal deliveries		All deliveries	
	F-values	Coefficients	F-values	Coefficients
Neckache				
Epidural	11.171	0.91403	7.4348	0.58520
Pethidine	5.208	0.62430	NS	NS
General anaesthesia	NS	NS	6.3156	0.52574
Primiparity	NS	NS	6.1929	0.53188
Shoulderache				
Longer 2nd stage labour	13.650	0.80118	NA	NA
Asian ethnic group	7.5755	0.59596	3.9161	0.35294
Section	NA	NA	12.840	0.64369
Primiparity	NS	NS	10.565	0.58199
Pain in arms				
Asian ethnic group	37.498	1.0000	42.404	0.89653
Section	NA		9.6212	0.42765
Pain in legs				
Asian ethnic group	34.004	0.79611	53.113	0.94287
Longer 1st stage labour	6.2257	0.34186	NA	NA
Younger age	5.0917	0.31012	NS	NA
Tranquilliser	4.3703	0.28535	6.9017	0.34056
Weakness in arms				
Asian ethnic group	69.936	0.95261	56.245	0.91731
Forceps	6.9164	0.30057	9.5647	0.44552
Weakness in legs				
Asian ethnic group	44.689	0.81634	48.160	0.83556
Non-married status	10.511	0.39689	11.541	0.40974
Pethidine	6.5689	0.33208	4.0196	0.24238
Forceps	4.6607	0.25506	NS	NS
General anaesthesia	NS	NS	6.5780	0.30974
Tingling hands/fingers				
Epidural	11.067	0.62052	10.984	0.83668
Pethidine	9.1645	0.55166	8.0977	0.71849
Heavier birthweight	8.7058	0.52697	NS	NS
Non-induced labour	6.6845	0.49134	NS	NS
High blood pressure	4.1947	0.38440	NS	NS

TABLE 10.6 – *continued*

| | Vaginal deliveries | | All deliveries | |
	F-values	Coefficients	F-values	Coefficients
Tingling feet/toes				
Forceps	6.3085	0.68384	6.7589	0.64064
PPH	5.3160	0.62778	NS	NS
Section	NA	NA	13.826*	0.91598

*If elective and emergency sections are included as two separate variables, emergency becomes significant (F-value = 10.586 Coefficient 0.88031) and elective is not quite significant.

or whether they were more evenly distributed. We found that 359 (68%) of the Asian women had no musculo-skeletal symptoms, while 104 had one symptom, 36 had two, and 31 reported more than two. The last group comprised only 11% of the symptomatic Asian women (Table 10.7, Panel A). We concluded that the musculo-skeletal symptoms were relatively widely distributed among the Asian women. A separate examination of pain and weakness in the arms and legs, confirmed this conclusion (Table 10.7, Panel B).

Parity, age and marital status

Primiparty was associated with neckache and shoulderache (above), and remained so after discriminant analysis (Table 10.5). These associations could have been generated by limiting 'acceptance' to new symptoms, with a consequent selective bias in favour of primiparous and younger women. We therefore carried out subsidiary discriminant analyses, which included symptom recurrences and continuations as well as new symptoms. The primiparity association disappeared completely, confirming that they were indeed artefacts.

The primary discriminant analysis showed associations with two other symptoms: early maternal age predicted pain in legs; and unmarried status predicted weakness in the legs (Table 10.5). Both factors are related to primiparity, and could also reflect biases arising from our inclusion criteria. Subsidiary discriminant analyses were again conducted for these symptoms,

TABLE 10.7

Musculo-skeletal symptoms and ethnic group

(a) All musculo-skeletal symptoms (headache; neckache; shoulderache; lower and middle backache; pain, weakness, tingling in arms and legs)

Number of symptoms	Asian (530)		Caucasian (10135)	
	No.	(%)	No.	(%)
None	359	(67.7)	8070	(79.6)
One	89	(16.8)	1336	(13.2)
Two	42	(7.9)	474	(4.7)
Three	17	(3.2)	150	(1.5)
Four	7	(1.3)	58	(0.6)
Five	4	(0.8)	22	(0.2)
Six	6	(1.1)	11	
Seven	4	(0.8)	8	
Eight	–		1	
Nine	1		5	
Ten	1		–	

(b) Pain in arms, legs – weakness in arms, legs

Number of symptoms	Asian		Caucasian	
	No.	(%)	No.	(%)
None	468	(88.3)	9784	(96.5)
One	34	(6.4)	263	(2.6)
Two	20	(3.8)	66	(0.7)
Three	4		13	
Four	4		9	

including both recurrences and new occurrences. The effect of early maternal age upon pain in the legs then disappeared, and was probably an artefact. The effect of unmarried status upon weakness in the legs, did not disappear. This may reflect more general fatigue associated with difficult domestic circumstances. We return to this point in a later chapter.

Obstetric and anaesthetic predictors

Epidural anaesthesia

Epidural anaesthesia was a primary focus of interest because of its strong relationships with backache and headache, and our suggested hypothesis in terms of a posturally related spinal-axis syndrome. Epidural anaesthesia had also exhibited crude associations with many of the musculo-skeletal symptoms (Table 10.1). Following discriminant analysis, epidural anaesthesia remained independently predictive of only two of them. These were neckache and tingling in the hands and fingers and, for both, an epidural was the dominant predictor (Table 10.6). Before accepting the possibility that neckache and tingling in the hands (like headache) might be additional 'optional' elements of the spinal axis syndrome, we examined the relationship further.

TABLE 10.8

Neckache and tingling in hands/fingers, epidural anaesthesia and 'normal' deliveries

	Neckache No. (%)	Tingling in hands No. (%)	Total women
'Normal' delivery with epidural	27 (2.46)	35 (3.19)	1098
'Normal' delivery no epidural	65 (1.40)	90 (1.94)	4646
'Abnormal' delivery with epidural	89 (2.43)	108 (2.94)	3668
'Abnormal' delivery no epidural	47 (2.05)	60 (2.62)	2289

Epidural anaesthesia, normal deliveries, neckache and tingling in hands

For backache and for headache we had tested and rejected the possibility that excess rates could result from the larger proportion of 'abnormal' deliveries among the epidurals. We repeated the exercise here, dividing the sample into 'normal' and 'abnormal' deliveries (as defined earlier) and measuring the effect of an epidural in each sub-group. This analysis is shown in Table 10.8 and a graphical representation is supplied in Figure 10.3. The findings both for neckache and for tingling in the hands resembled those for headache. In 'abnormal' deliveries an epidural made little additional difference to the already-raised symptom-rate, but among the 'normal' deliveries there was a significant association. There was therefore no evidence that the increased rates after an epidural might have resulted indirectly from the relationship between the procedure and the less straightforward deliveries.

Figure 10.3 Neck/Hands, Epidurals & 'Normal' Births

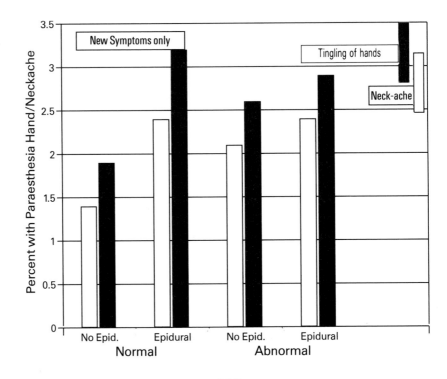

Epidural anaesthesia and Caesarean section

With backache, an epidural given for an elective Caesarean section was not associated with an increased symptom risk. With headache, an epidural caused no symptom increase after either form of section: just after vaginal delivery. Table 10.9 shows a similar analysis for neckache and for tingling in the hands. In each case the significant epidural excess was limited to vaginal deliveries: as it had been for headache.

TABLE 10.9

	Neckache No. (%)	Tingling in hands No. (%)	Total women
Neckache, tingling in hands/fingers, epidural anaesthesia and type of delivery			
Vaginal with epidural	86 (2.33)	110 (2.98)	3688
Vaginal no epidural	91 (1.51)	130 (2.13)	6098
Elective with epidural	9 (2.11)	9 (2.11)	426
Elective no epidural	11 (3.20)	8 (2.33)	344
Emergency with epidural	21 (3.22)	24 (3.68)	652
Emergency no epidural	9 (1.83)	12 (2.43)	493

Extensions of the 'spinal axis syndrome'?

Neckache and tingling in the hands, the primary musculo-skeletal correlates of epidural anaesthesia, are related to each other in neuro-anatomical terms. There were 46 women who reported both symptoms, with an Odds Ratio of 11.5. The relationship with epidural anaesthesia might be primary for one symptom, and secondary for the other. To test this, separate discriminant analyses of each symptom were conducted, holding the other symptom as an independent variable. In each case the independent predictive effect of the epidural anaesthesia was retained. In separate detailed tabulations (Table 10.10) the greatest effect of an epidural was upon the combination of neckache and tingling in the hands (RR = 2.27), although the numbers in this group were small.

TABLE 10.10

Combinations of neckache, tingling in hands/fingers and epidural anaesthesia

	Neckache alone No. (%)	Tingling alone No. (%)	Both symptoms No. (%)	Total women
Epidural	88 (1.85)	115 (2.41)	28 (0.59)	4766
No epidural	94 (1.36)	132 (1.90)	18 (0.26)	6935
Relative risks	1.36	1.26	2.27	

TABLE 10.11

'Symptom combinations' and epidural anaesthesia

Symptom combinations	Epidural No. (%)	No epidural No. (%)	Relative risks	Total women
Headache alone*	124 (2.60)	156 (2.25)	1.16	280
Neckache alone	34 (0.71)	45 (0.65)	1.09	79
Backache alone**	735 (15.52)	614 (8.85)	1.74	1349
Tingling hands alone	70 (1.47)	89 (1.28)	1.15	159
Head and neckache	12 (0.25)	9 (0.13)	1.92	21
Head and backache	85 (1.78)	44 (0.63)	2.83	129
Head and tingling hands	10 (0.21)	13 (0.19)	1.11	23
Neck and backache	30 (0.63)	30 (0.43)	1.47	60
Neck and tingling hands	11 (0.23)	10 (0.14)	1.64	21
Back and tingling hands	26 (0.55)	24 (0.35)	1.57	50
Head, neck and backache	14 (0.29)	11 (0.16)	1.81	25
Head, neck and tingling	1	–		1
Head, back and tingling	14 (0.29)	8 (0.12)	2.42	22
Neck, back and tingling	9 (0.19)	6 (0.09)	2.11	15
All four	7 (0.15)	4 (0.06)	2.50	9
None of these	3584 (75.2)	5769 (83.2)	0.90	9353
Total symptoms	1453	1255		
Mean	0.30	0.18	1.67	
Total women	4766 (100)	6935 (100)		

*'Headache' refers to frequent headaches and migraine
**'Backache' refers to all backache: middle, lower or both

Combinations of neckache, tingling in the hands, backache and headache were cross-tabulated against epidural anaesthesia (Table 10.11). Overall, the total numbers of reports of all these symptoms averaged 0.30 among women who had an epidural and 0.18 after a non-epidural delivery: a 60% increase. For some of the symptom combinations the numbers were small, so precise conclusions are difficult, but the epidural association did appear to be selective. Apart from backache, none of the solitary symptoms showed an enhanced epidural risk; nor generally did those symptom combinations which did not include backache. The epidural relationship was mainly limited to a 'spinal-axis syndrome' consisting either of backache alone, or backache combined with one or more of the three other symptoms.

General anaesthesia and Caesarean sections

Almost all general anaesthesias (97%) were given for Caesarean sections, so it is difficult to separate any associations of the two procedures. This is especially true for low frequency symptoms, where the small numbers did not permit comprehensive multi-way tabulations. However, general anaesthesia was shown to be a predictor of neckache and Caesarean section of shoulderache and pain in the arms. There are obvious anatomical relationships between these three symptoms. Epidural anaesthesia, the alternative form of anaesthesia for sections, was shown to be an overall predictor of neckache after vaginal deliveries, but symptoms rates were not significantly raised after a section (see earlier and Table 10.9). Excess neckache after a Caesarean delivery was therefore more likely to be related to general anaesthesia. An explanation is suggested later.

General anaesthesia also predicted weakness in the legs; and Caesarean section, tingling in the feet or toes. Again there are possible anatomical and neurological connections between the two symptoms, although whether Caesarean section or general anaesthesia is dominant cannot be determined by this data set.

Other obstetric predictors

Forceps delivery was an independent predictor of weakness in the legs, weakness in the arms, and tingling in the feet or toes, and for the latter it was the dominant predictor (Table 10.6). After a forceps delivery, 1.43% of women reported tingling, compared with 0.78% in vaginal deliveries without forceps (RR = 1.81); 1.56% reported weakness in the legs compared with 1.08% (RR = 1.44); and 1.69% reported weakness in the arms compared with 1.14% (RR = 1.48).

A long first stage of labour was the dominant predictor of pain in the legs. It was more than twice as frequent when the first stage lasted six hours or more, as when it lasted under two hours (RR = 2.21). The use of tranquillisers during labour also predicted pain in the legs, with a relative risk of 1.70. Pethidine used for pain relief predicted neckache and tingling in the hands, two related symptoms, as well as weakness in the legs. We consider pethidine further in Chapter 16.

Tingling in the hands was associated with greater birthweight, with a non-induced labour, and with pregnancy hypertension. Cross-tabulation (Table 10.12) showed that the birthweight relationship was confined to the epidural deliveries. The association with non-induced labour is difficult to explain, but is comparable with a similar finding for backache.

TABLE 10.12

Tingling in hands/fingers, epidural anaesthesia and birthweight

	Tingling in hands No. (%)	Total women
Epidural		
Up to 3200 grams	45 (2.55)	1762
3201 – 3700 grams	50 (2.77)	1807
3701 grams or more	48 (4.01)	1197
No epidural		
Up to 3200 grams	52 (1.99)	2618
3201 – 3700 grams	60 (2.18)	2750
3701 grams or more	38 (2.43)	1567

Discussion

Musculo-skeletal symptoms (excluding backache and headache) were each reported by relatively small proportions of women; but together they amounted to 1548 separately recorded symptoms. One in twelve women reported one or more of them. Within this overall picture we found a complex matrix of inter-correlations, and several different patterns of association with external determinants. The full picture is difficult to interpret, but several constellations emerged.

The first was an extension of the spinal-axis syndrome postulated in earlier chapters. This now appears as a complex group of symptoms, of which backache is an obligatory component, but which is variable supplemented by headache, by neckache, and by tingling in the hands or fingers. The primary mechanism might be postural but the incidence is enhanced – almost doubled – by epidural anaesthesia. Although epidurals showed additional crude statistical associations with shoulder ache, pains in the arms and tingling in the feet, these disappeared on standardisation. Musculo-skeletal symptoms other than backache-associated headache, neckache and tingling in the hands, are probably not part of this syndrome.

The excess rates of the different musculo-skeletal symptoms among the Asian women corresponded inexactly with the ancillary components of the spinal-axis syndrome as already proposed. We considered the possibility of other (possibly overlapping) explanations for this striking excess of skeletal symptoms among Asians, especially pains and weakness in the limbs. The most obvious hypothesis concerns the types of nutritional deficiencies typically found in Asian women, (Brooke et al 1980; Sturman and Beevers 1990; Wharton and Wharton 1989) and a consequent latent osteomalacia. Pre-existing deficiencies of calcium and of vitamin D, and the additional metabolic and physical stresses of pregnancy and delivery, may be enough in some women to produce symptomatic osteomalacia. This hypothesis is in urgent need of testing especially since, if it is upheld, the extensive skeletal problems of the Asian women have potential solutions.

There was some evidence that there might be at least one other form of postural injury, separate from the epidural associated syndrome, although affecting only small numbers of women. Caesarean section and general anaesthesia, themselves closely associated, were jointly or separately predictive of neckache, shoulder ache, and pains in the arms. These symptoms were inter-correlated in statistical terms and are relatable in anatomical terms. They arise, plausibly, from the postures and manipulations associated with Caesarean section, especially under general anaesthesia, where they are unprotected by muscle tone, and where the neck is positioned to facilitate intubation. In Chapter 9 we also recorded excess rates of headache after Caesarean section under general anaesthesia, possibly arising through the same mechanisms. Overall, the skeletal/ligamentous system of the parturient women seems to be extraordinarily/sensitive.

The question next arises what other patterns of association might remain when these two layers described above have been peeled away. The main unexplained residual associations included a relationship between pethidine and subsequent neckache, tingling in the hands and weakness in the legs; and another between general anaesthesia and weakness in the legs – without the explanatory mediation of backache, and not easily linked with the mechanically-related neck/shoulder syndrome. There was also a pattern of weakness in the legs and arms, and tingling in the feet and toes, associated with forceps delivery: and pains in the legs associated with a long first stage, and the use of tranquillisers during early labour; tingling in the hands associated with a large baby; and tingling in the feet associated with a Caesarean section.

Some of the difficulties of interpretation could have arisen because the situation is indeed intrinsically complex, with relatively small numbers of women affected, and its resolution fundamentally beyond the capabilities of the simple data assembled for the task. Furthermore, some of the reported symptoms could be the result of psychological rather than physical trauma. However other postulates could be ischaemic neurological injuries from intra-pelvic pressure or possible peripheral-neuritic sensitivity reactions to drugs. We shall have occasion to raise these issues in a later chapter.

Chapter 11 – Bladder Problems: Stress Incontinence and Urinary Frequency

The questionnaire asked two questions on bladder problems. One was about stress incontinence, specified as 'hard to hold urine when jump, sneeze, etc'. The other was about urinary frequency, described as 'pass urine very often'.

Frequency of occurrence

Stress incontinence, starting for the first time within three months of delivery, and lasting longer than six weeks, was reported by 1782 women (15.2%); and urinary frequency was reported by 668 (5.7%). Within each group, 416 had experienced both symptoms; 2034 women (17.4%) had suffered either stress incontinence or urinary frequency or both.

An additional 637 women (5.4%) reported stress incontinence within three months of delivery, and lasting more than six weeks, but not as a new symptom; bringing the total to 2419 (20.6%). An additional 438 (3.7%) reported urinary frequency as a continuation or recurrence, bringing the total for this symptom to 1106 (9.4%). Overall, there were more new bladder symptoms than recurrences. Among all the women reporting long term stress incontinence within three months, 73% said it was a new problem: and for urinary frequency, 58%. But after a first baby, 90% said it was new: and 74% for urinary frequency. The association between childbirth and these bladder symptoms, especially stress incontinence, is highly specific.

In addition to these totals, many women could not adequately date their symptoms – 619 in the case of stress incontinence and 390 for urinary frequency. All were reported as occurring after the index delivery but the women had either not given the onset date, or the duration, or had not said whether it had occurred before. These items were all required in order to fulfil the criteria for inclusion within the main analysis, and all these cases were therefore excluded. The true prevalences must therefore be greater than the estimates based on fully dated reports.

We did not ask about the specific circumstances in which previous bladder symptoms had arisen, but many women volunteered the information. In 131 of the 637 cases of recurring stress incontinence (21%), and in 54 of the 438 cases of recurring urinary frequency (12%), the women added on the questionnaire a note that it had started after a previous delivery. In a further 64 of the 637 cases of recurrent stress incontinence and 48 of the 438 cases of recurrent urinary frequency (11%), they noted that the symptoms had begun during the pregnancy prior to the delivery itself, failing thus to meet the strict criteria for inclusion within the main affected groups.

The main analyses were limited to the 1782 fully dated cases of new post-delivery stress incontinence, and the 668 fully dated cases of new post-delivery urinary frequency so that we could relate them to the recorded circumstances and procedures of the delivery in question. Because it seemed possible (as with headache) that the predictors of urinary frequency and those of stress incontinence might differ, we conducted our first analyses for each of these bladder symptoms separately, and examined the combinations later.

Durations and onsets

Few of these bladder problems were transient. Only 8% of women with stress incontinence were clear of it after three months; 75% had it for over a year, and 70% still had it at the time of questioning. Of the women with urinary frequency, only 6% had it for less than three months, 81% had it for more than a year, and 75% said that they still had it.

Both bladder symptoms began very soon after delivery. Of the 1782 cases of stress incontinence, 85% (1517) started within the first post-partum week, and 93% (1658) within four weeks. For urinary frequency, 82% (549) began in the first week and 92% (615) within four weeks. The proportions reporting immediate onsets were much greater than for backache or for headache/migraine.

We examined the onset distributions of all new cases of long term stress incontinence and urinary frequency, within the whole of the first post-partum year, including those otherwise excluded as beyond the three month limit. The first year total for new stress incontinence was 1869, of which 1517 (81%) had started within a week of delivery, 1658 (89%) within four weeks and 1782 (95%) within three months. For urinary frequency, the full year total was 722, of which 549 (76%) started within a week of delivery, 85% (615) within four weeks, and 93% (668) within three months. These timings confirm that both of these bladder symptoms are associated very specifically with the delivery of a child.

Medical consultation

The doctor was seldom consulted about either of these bladder symptoms. Only 14% of women with stress incontinence and 22% of those with urinary frequency had consulted their general practitioners. Where both symptoms were present, 24% had consulted. As with double reports of middle and lower backache, and of headache and migraine, the combined occurrences may be an indicator of severity but if so, this had little effect upon consultation rates. Low levels of general practitioner consultation for stress incontinence (not specifically following childbirth) were also noted in studies by Jolleys (1988) and by Yarnell et al. (1981).

In contrast with backache and headache, the durations of the bladder problems did raise the frequency of medical consultation. The doctor was consulted for 8% of those (few) cases of stress incontinence lasting less than a year, but for 16% of cases lasting more than two years. For urinary frequency the corresponding proportions were 16% and 24%.

For stress incontinence (but not urinary frequency) medical consultation rates were also influenced by parity and by the mother's age. The doctor was consulted by 11% of the primiparous women with stress incontinence compared with 15% of multiparous women; and by 11% of those under 25, compared with 19% of those aged 35 or more.

We asked the women about treatment. Of the 249 who had consulted their doctor with stress incontinence, 49% said they had been given treatment; and 39% of those consulting with urinary frequency. Many women said that the treatment, particularly for stress incontinence, consisted of advice about exercises to strengthen perineal muscles. Hospital referral rates from among those who had consulted were relatively high: for stress incontinence 25% were referred for specialist advice: 32% for frequency. Nevertheless these referrals represented only 3.5% and 7.0% of the total number sho had reported each of the symptoms. Women who reported both bladder symptoms had higher rates of specialist referral, 37% of those consulting.

Factors associated with stress incontinence

Many different factors were associated with stress incontinence. First there were strong associations with the social and demographic characteristics of the mothers, shown in the upper part of Table 11.1 and in Figure 11.1. (Figure 11.2 shows the analogous relationships for urinary frequency.) Stress incontinence was more frequent in primiparae, in older, and in married women. Women in social classes I and II, taller women, and Caucasians also reported higher rates. Second, there were many associations with obstetric and anaesthetic events, as set out in the lower panels of Table 11.1. Stress incontinence was more frequent following occipito-posterior fetal presentations and after longer first and second stages of labour; also with epidural anaesthesia, forceps, episiotomy, perineal laceration, heavier babies, longer babies and babies with a greater head circumference. Symptom rates were significantly lower following Caesarean section – elective or emergency – and following pre-term delivery.

TABLE 11.1

Characteristics associated with bladder problems*

	Stress incontinence No. (%)	Urinary frequency No. (%)	Total women
Whole sample	1782 (15.2)	668 (5.7)	11701
Parity 0	712 (17.0)	276 (6.6)	4185
1	732 (15.7)	260 (5.6)	4669
2+	338 (11.9)	132 (4.6)	2847
Under 25 years	331 (12.6)	156 (5.9)	2625
25 – 29	636 (15.1)	234 (5.5) NS	4225
30 or more	815 (16.8)	278 (5.7)	4851
Married	1635 (15.5)	597 (5.7) NS	10525
Single/Div/Wid/Sep	147 (12.5)	71 (6.0)	1176
Social class I & II	508 (17.6)	148 (5.1) NS	2882
III, IV & V	1064 (15.1)	424 (6.0)	7048
Caucasian	1619 (16.0)	604 (6.0)	10135
Asian	39 (7.4)	19 (3.6)	530
Height under 150 cms	33 (11.5)	17 (5.9)	286
150 – 159 cms	536 (14.4)	219 (5.9) NS	3718
160 – 169 cms	908 (15.6)	338 (5.8)	5829
170 cms or more	208 (18.8)	59 (5.3)	1104
Occipito-Anterior	1581 (15.4)	586 (5.7)	10265
Occipito-Posterior	88 (17.1)	35 (6.8) NS	514
Other presentations	113 (12.3)	47 (5.1)	916
First stage labour			
Under 2 hours	284 (13.8)	95 (4.6)	2054
2 – 5 hrs 59 mins	895 (17.0)	326 (6.2)	5264
6 – 9 hrs 59 mins	291 (17.3)	100 (5.9)	1684
10 hours or more	92 (18.0)	39 (7.6)	511
Second stage			
Up to 15 minutes	389 (12.9)	136 (4.5)	3014
16 – 30 minutes	334 (12.9)	129 (6.0)	2142
30 – 59 minutes	307 (17.6)	95 (5.4)	1749
60 – 119 minutes	351 (18.9)	140 (7.5)	1858
120 minutes or more	210 (22.4)	73 (7.8)	939

TABLE 11.1 Cont.

	Stress incontinence No. (%)	Urinary frequency No. (%)	Total women
Rotational forceps	106 (23.9)	34 (7.7)	443
Straight forceps	362 (19.5)	139 (7.5)	1858
No forceps	1314 (14.0)	495 (5.3)	9400
Vaginal delivery	1603 (16.4)	572 (5.8)	9785
Elective section	69 (9.0)	33 (4.3) NS	770
Emergency section	110 (9.6)	63 (5.5)	1145
Episiotomy	898 (17.6)	320 (6.3)	5112
Laceration	483 (16.6)	159 (5.5) NS	2907
Intact perineum	416 (11.1)	191 (5.1)	3729
Epidural	779 (16.3)	368 (5.3)	6935
Non-epidural	1003 (14.5)	300 (6.3)	4766
Pudendal block	54 (19.0)	23 (8.1)	284
No pudendal block	1728 (15.1)	645 (5.6)	11417
Pre-term gestation	89 (11.1)	39 (4.9) NS	800
Term gestation	1693 (15.5)	629 (5.8)	10901
Birthweight			
Up to 2500 grams	73 (9.5)	35 (4.6)	767
2501 – 3200 grams	521 (14.4)	211 (5.8)	3613
3201 – 3700 grams	697 (15.3)	226 (5.0)	4557
3701 grams or more	491 (17.8)	196 (7.1)	2764
Head circumference			
Up to 30 cms	26 (8.9)	18 (6.2)	291
31 – 33 cms	410 (14.5)	156 (5.5) NS	2835
34 – 35 cms	917 (15.2)	330 (5.5)	6044
36 cms or more	423 (17.2)	159 (6.4)	2495
Length			
Up to 47cms	152 (13.4)	72 (5.4)	1336
48 – 52 cms	957 (15.1)	355 (5.6) NS	6356
53 cms or more	656 (17.2)	228 (6.0)	3809

*Symptoms starting within three months of delivery, never previously experienced, lasting longer than six weeks.

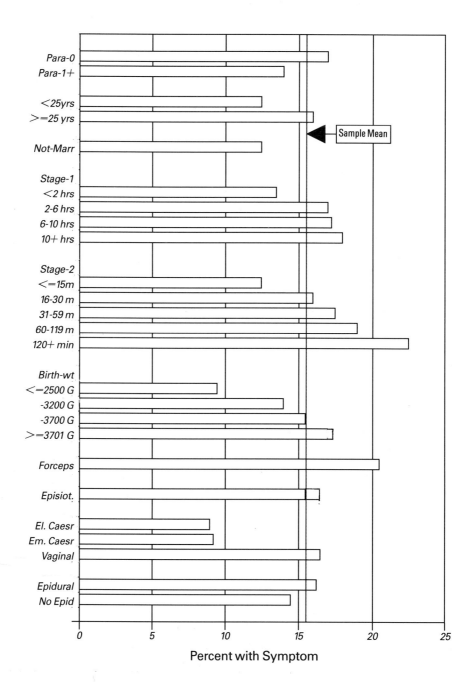

Figure 11.1

Stress Incontinence & Associated Factors

Primary predictors of stress incontinence and secondary associations

Many of the social factors and the obstetric circumstances and events were themselves inter-related. We had to disentangle those which were independent primary predictors from those which were only indirectly associated with stress incontinence. Discriminant analysis takes simultaneous account of all factors, and the results are shown in Table 11.2. The first two columns refer to vaginal deliveries, and the last two show the results of vaginal and Caesarean deliveries together, but at the cost of discarding durations of labour as potential factors. These analyses showed that the dominant social predictors of stress incontinence were primiparity, higher maternal age and (to a lesser extent) social class I and II. Asian ethnic group was a significant negative predictor. The crude associations with marital status and maternal height disappeared; they must have been secondary associations.

TABLE 11.2

Discriminant analysis of characteristics associated with stress incontinence

	Vaginal deliveries		All deliveries	
	F value	Coefficients	F value	Coefficients
Primiparity	22.657	0.48013	24.614	0.3991
Increasing age	26.859	0.47372	29.830	0.37672
Heavier birthweight	24.073	0.42065	15.667	0.27348
Longer 2nd stage labour	15.789	0.3775	N/A	N/A
Non-Asian ethnic group	14.935	0.32507	17.679	0.29297
Social class I, II	6.655	0.22191	17.819	0.28358
No section	N/A	N/A	35.242	0.45486
Forceps	N.S.	N.S.	20.296	0.34855
Laceration	N.S.	N.S.	5.257	0.17069

There were also two dominant positive obstetric predictors: greater birthweight, and a longer second stage of labour. Caesarean section was a significant negative predictor. Forceps delivery and perineal laceration emerged as significant predictors only in the discriminant analysis of all deliveries, possibly because duration of labour was omitted from the analysis, so that forceps then probably served as a proxy for this missing variable.

In the following paragraphs we consider each of the independent symptom predictors in more detail, looking first at the social factors and then at the obstetric ones.

Social predictors

Parity and age

We considered first the joint age and parity relationships. Interpretations for these factors are always complicated by the 'first-time' inclusion criterion, as discussed in earlier chapters. This results in the systematic exclusion of many affected multiparous and older women, since they are more likely to have had symptoms before. In the case of stress incontinence, however, the maternal age association was in the opposite direction to that expected from this cause; there was more first-time stress incontinence in **older** women. This association is almost certainly real: and indeed likely to be stronger than the analysis suggests.

To examine this further, we conducted additional discriminant analyses for all symptoms beginning within three months of delivery and lasting more than six weeks, but **irrespective** of previous occurrence. The association with mothers' age was strengthened, confirming our supposition, and the association with primiparity disappeared. Additional discriminant analyses were also conducted in primiparae and in multiparae separately. Increasing maternal age remained as a major independent predictor within each of these parity groups. We tabulated the age relationship for stress incontinence within each separate parity group, (Table 11.3) again confirming its consistency (Column 1). Column two of Table 11.3 shows further tabulations for the various parities, incorporating women who had also stress incontinence before. The age gradient is seen clearly everywhere.

Table 11.3 also confirmed the supposition that the diminishing risk of first time incontinence with increasing parity was indeed an artefact of progressive exclusion from candidature. The all-ages prevalences of newly occurring symptoms (Column 1) declined with increasing parity, but when the previous occurrence exclusion rule was not applied, (Column 2) there was no such decline. The pattern was repeated in several individual age bands.

TABLE 11.3

Stress incontinence, maternal age and parity

	Stress incontinence No. (%)	Stress incontinence, irrespective of previous history No. (%)	Total women
Parity 0			
Age 24 or less	211 (13.5)	238 (15.3)	1558
25 – 29	275 (18.0)	311 (20.4)	1527
30 or more	226 (20.6)	244 (22.2)	1100
All ages	712 (17.0)	793 (18.9)	4185
Parity 1			
Age 24 or less	104 (12.7)	139 (17.0)	819
25 – 29	276 (14.8)	379 (20.4)	1860
30 or more	352 (17.7)	504 (25.3)	1990
All ages	732 (15.7)	1024 (21.9)	4669
Parity 2			
Age 24 or less	12 (6.0)	29 (14.4)	201
25 – 29	68 (10.4)	113 (17.3)	654
30 or more	162 (14.4)	290 (25.8)	1123
All ages	246 (12.4)	432 (21.8)	1978
Parity 3+			
Age 24 or less	4 (8.5)	6 (12.8)	47
25 – 29	17 (9.2)	25 (13.6)	184
30 or more	71 (11.1)	139 (21.8)	638
All ages	92 (10.6)	170 (19.6)	869

TABLE 11.4

Stress incontinence, maternal age, birthweight and duration of second stage labour

Duration of second stage	Age up to 24 yrs		25-29 years		30 years or more		All ages	
	Stress incontinence No. (%)	Total women	Stress incontinence No. (%)	Total women	Stress incontinence No. (%)	Total women	Stress incontinence No. (%)	Total women
Birthweight up to 3200 grams								
Up to 15 mins	28 (11.1)	253	49 (11.4)	428	52 (11.4)	448	128 (11.3)	1129
16 – 59 mins	48 (11.5)	419	69 (13.2)	521	92 (17.6)	523	209 (14.3)	1463
60 – 119 mins	25 (14.0)	179	38 (17.7)	215	40 (17.7)	227	102 (16.7)	621
120 mins or more	10 (15.2)	69	27 (24.1)	112	32 (34.4)	92	67 (25.3)	273
All durations	111 (12.1)	920	183 (14.3)	1276	216 (16.7)	1290	510 (14.6)	3486
Birthweight 3201 – 3700 grams								
Up to 15 mins	17 (7.8)	219	59 (13.0)	455	81 (14.8)	546	157 (12.9)	1220
16 – 59 mins	47 (13.4)	352	93 (16.7)	556	116 (18.5)	624	256 (16.7)	1532
60 – 119 mins	29 (13.1)	222	56 (19.2)	291	64 (24.6)	258	149 (19.3)	771
120 mins or more	15 (14.0)	107	30 (20.0)	150	28 (22.4)	129	73 (18.9)	386
All durations	108 (12.0)	900	238 (16.4)	1452	289 (18.6)	1557	635 (16.2)	3909

TABLE 11.4 – *continued*

Stress incontinence, maternal age, birthweight and duration of second stage labour

Duration of second stage	Age up to 24 yrs		25-29 years		30 years or more		All ages	
	Stress incontinence No. (%)	Total women	Stress incontinence No. (%)	Total women	Stress incontinence No. (%)	Total women	Stress incontinence No. (%)	Total women
Birthweight 3701 grams or more								
Up to 15 mins	13 (14.1)	92	37 (15.4)	240	53 (15.9)	333	103 (15.5)	665
16 – 59 mins	30 (17.1)	175	66 (20.2)	326	80 (20.3)	395	176 (19.6)	896
60 – 119 mins	23 (21.9)	105	35 (18.3)	191	41 (24.1)	170	99 (21.2)	466
120 mins or more	25 (30.1)	83	20 (20.0)	100	23 (23.7)	97	68 (24.3)	280
All durations	91 (20.0)	455	158 (18.4)	857	197 (19.8)	995	446 (19.3)	2307
All weights								
Up to 15 mins	58 (10.3)	564	145 (12.9)	1123	186 (14.0)	1327	388 (12.9)	3014
16 – 59 mins	125 (13.2)	946	228 (16.3)	1403	205 (13.3)	1542	641 (16.5)	3891
60 – 119 mins	77 (15.2)	506	129 (18.5)	697	145 (22.1)	655	350 (18.8)	1858
120 mins or more	50 (19.3)	259	77 (21.3)	362	83 (26.1)	318	208 (22.2)	939
All durations	310 (13.6)	2275	579 (16.2)	3585	619 (16.1)	3842	1590 (16.4)	9702

Ethnic group and social class

Asian women reported must less stress incontinence that Caucasians (Table 11.1). This might have been secondary to an age effect, since the Asians were younger, but the difference remained after the discriminant analysis had taken account of this and other confounding factors (Table 11.2). The crude relative risk of stress incontinence in Asians was 0.46 compared with Caucasians. We wondered whether this difference might arise from language difficulties and consequent reporting bias, or some other cultural difference of understanding or willingness to report symptoms. If so then the reporting problems are symptom-specific, because there were no such parallels for backache, headache and musculo-skeletal symptoms. However, the questions relating to stress incontinence (see Questionnaire, Appendix 1) might be more difficult to comprehend and are of a more personal nature, so the possibility of symptom-specific reporting differences remains.

The positive association between stress incontinence and social classes I and II might also have reflected indirect associations with parity and maternal age. However, the subsidiary discriminant analysis which also included women with the continuing and recurring symptoms, retained the association. Social class remained as an independent predictor and could not be discarded as a selective artefact. However symptom-specific response-biases between different social groups, analogous to those discussed above for Asians, may offer a partial explanation.

Obstetric and anaesthetic predictors

Duration of second stage labour and birthweight

A longer second stage of labour and the delivery of a heavier baby were both independent predictors of stress incontinence. They were themselves inter-related, and each was associated with maternal age, although in opposite directions; long second stage labours were less frequent, and heavier babies more frequent, in older women.

We tried to localise the effects of these variations to particular sub-sets of the population. Table 11.4 tabulates the joint relationships (among vaginal deliveries) of combinations of maternal ages, birthweights and durations of the second stage. The effects of a prolonged second stage could not be localised to particular sub-groups; increased rates of stress incontinence were observed in

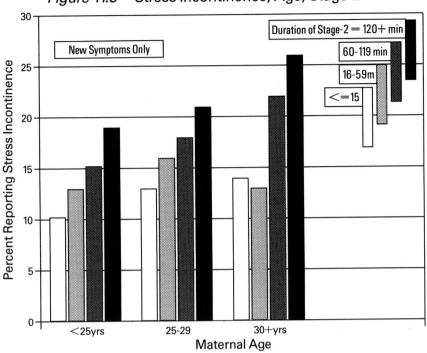

Figure 11.3   Stress Incontinence, Age, Stage-2

all age groups (see Figure 11.3) and at all birthweights. It was the most consistent predictor. The other two factors produced less striking and less consistent associations, and they seemed to interact with each other. Thus the age association was limited to women with lower birthweight infants of 3700 grams or less: a large infant seemed to counter-balance the effect of increasing age. The weight association was most marked in younger women and only evident in older women who had short labours. Increasing birthweight and increasing age behaved to some extent as alternative predictors. The general effects of all these predictors were not simply additive, which might suggest that there could be more than one mechanism at work.

Caesarean section

Stress incontinence was much less frequent after a Caesarean section than after vaginal delivery (RR = 0.57). The 'protective' effect was similar for both elective and emergency Caesareans suggesting that a major component of the risk is mediated by the vaginal passage of the infant. Even after a Caesarean section, however, stress incontinence sometimes occurred: among those who had a section, almost one in ten (9.3%) reported subsequent new long-term stress incontinence.

In order to dissect the possible mechanisms further, we conducted additional discriminant analysis and constructed sub-tabulations, only for women who had had a Caesarean section (Table 11.5). The discriminant analysis revealed only one significant predictor of stress incontinence after a Caesarean delivery: greater maternal age. The association with increasing age was the same among Caesareans as among vaginal deliveries (see Figure 11.4). Increased birthweight with a Caesarean delivery however did not raise the risk. Detailed tabulations (Table 11.5) confirmed these relationships.

Duration of second stage labour and forceps

Discriminant analysis of all delivery types, vaginal and Caesarean sections together, appeared to incriminate the use of forceps as a predictor of stress incontinence (Table 11.2, Column 2), but this was not confirmed in the analysis

TABLE 11.5

Stress incontinence, maternal age and birthweight in Caesarean sections

	Age Up to 24 yrs		25-29 years		30 years or more	
Birthweight	Stress incontin-ence No. (%)	Total women	Stress incontin-ence No. (%)	Total women	Stress incontin-ence No. (%)	Total women
Up to 3100 grams	6 (4.8)	124	22 (9.5)	231	46 (11.5)	399
3101 – 3600 grams	7 (6.4)	109	18 (9.3)	193	33 (10.6)	310
3601 grams or more	6 (6.1)	99	13 (7.0)	185	28 (10.7)	262
All weights	19 (5.7)	332	53 (8.7)	609	107 (11.0)	971

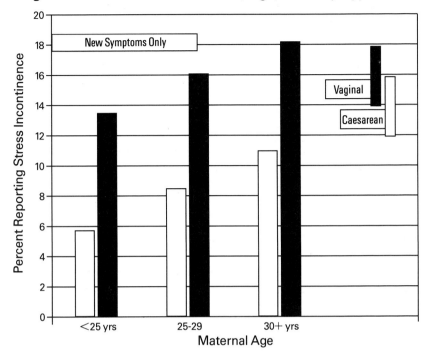

Figure 11.4 Stress Incontinence, Age, Delivery-Type

of vaginal deliveries alone. We have suggested that it could be an artefact arising because forceps was acting as a proxy for a long labour. Table 11.1 had shown a crude difference between the two types of forceps, rotational forceps being associated with higher symptom rates. An additional discriminant analysis conducted for vaginal deliveries, but entering the two types of forceps separately, did show rotational but not straight forceps to be a significant predictor of stress incontinence ($F = 5.9888$).

Since the forceps/second stage relationship was clearly complex, we tabulated them jointly, also examining each parity groups and each type of forceps separately. The results are shown in Table 11.6. This demonstrated that rates after rotational forceps were generally high, but straight forceps exhibited a highly localised predictive relationship, limited to multiparae delivering after a second stage of more than one hour. Duration of an hour or more in multiparae is sufficiently unusual to suggest that its combination with forceps may represent the presence of complex additional 'uncoded' hazards of an especially traumatic delivery.

TABLE 11.6

Stress incontinence, duration of second stage labour and forceps in vaginal deliveries

Duration of second stage	No forceps		Straight Forceps		Rotational forceps	
	Stress incontinence No. (%)	Total women	Stress incontinence No. (%)	Total women	Stress incontinence No. (%)	Total women
Primiparae						
Up to 15 mins	22 (13.5)	161	10 (19.6)	51	1	9
16 – 59 mins	170 (17.6)	969	42 (17.1)	246	12 (21.8)	55
60 – 119 mins	114 (19.0)	606	77 (15.6)	494	34 (32.4)	105
120 mins or more	36 (23.1)	158	96 (23.4)	411	32 (25.2)	127
Multiparae						
Up to 15 mins	348 (12.8)	2720	7 (10.3)	68	1	5
16 – 59 mins	375 (15.8)	2366	33 (15.7)	210	9 (20.0)	45
60 – 119 mins	55 (14.4)	383	65 (29.4)	221	6 (12.2)	49
120 mins or more	14 (16.0)	87	23 (19.3)	119	9 (24.3)	37

What predicts onsets and durations of stress incontinence?

The analyses described above were limited to first-time stress incontinence, which had started within three months of delivery and lasted more than six weeks. However, as part of a search for etiological heterogeneities we conducted separate analyses for symptoms beginning at different times, and with different durations. The results for different onsets are given in Table 11.7 and for different durations, in Table 11.8.

Table 11.7 confirms the high proportions of stress incontinence with immediate onset. It also demonstrates that the associations with increased birthweight, a long second stage, the localised effects of forceps delivery (not shown) and vaginal delivery were limited to the symptoms starting within a week of delivery. Symptoms beginning two to thirteen weeks after delivery were related only to maternal age. Separate discriminant analyses of first week and later onsets (2-13 weeks) confirmed that while all the above factors predicted the first week cases, only increased maternal age predicted the later ones.

Table 11.8 shows differing durations of symptoms and the relationships with the main predictors. It confirmed the high proportion (70%) of new symptoms still persisting at the time of our enquiry. Discriminant analysis of these 'chronic' symptoms re-confirmed the importance of all the main predictive factors already described, but the rankings changed. Maternal age was the dominant predictor of the persistent symptoms. In a comparable discriminant analysis of symptoms which had eventually subsided, maternal age was no longer significant. For this group, prolonged second stage was the most powerful predictor.

Factors associated with urinary frequency

The factors that were associated with the second bladder symptom, urinary frequency are shown in Table 11.1 and in Figure 11.2. They were less impressive than for stress incontinence. The only socially defined group of women with an increased rate of new post-partum urinary frequency were primiparae; and the only group with a significantly reduced rate were the Asian women. In contrast with stress incontinence, increasing maternal age was not associated.

The lower part of Table 11.1 shows associations with obstetric and anaesthetic factors. They were similar to, but less powerful than, those for stress incontinence. Epidural anaesthesia, pudendal block, longer labours, forceps deliveries and heavier babies were all significantly associated with higher rates of urinary frequency. In contrast to stress incontinence, there was no reduction following a Caesarean section.

TABLE 11.7

Differing onsets of stress incontinence, age, birthweight, second stage labour and type of delivery

	Onset Within 1 week	2-13 weeks	Between 3-12 months	Total women
	No. (%)	No. (%)	No. (%)	
Maternal age				
Up to 24 years	282 (10.74)	49 (1.87)	14 (0.53)	2625
25 – 29 years	547 (12.95)	89 (2.11)	36 (0.83)	4225
30 yrs or more	688 (14.18)	127 (2.62)	37 (0.76)	4851
Relative risks	1.32	1.40	1.43(NS)	
Birthweight				
Up to 3200 grams	493 (11.26)	101 (2.31)	33 (0.75)	4380
3201 – 3700 grams	588 (12.90)	109 (2.39)	26 (0.57)	4557
3701 grams or more	436 (15.77)	55 (1.99)	28 (1.01)	2764
Relative risks	1.40	0.86(NS)	1.35(NS)	
Duration of second stage labour (vaginal deliveries only)				
Under 60 mins	873 (12.64)	157 (2.27)	59 (0.85)	6905
60 mins or more	487 (17.41)	74 (2.65)	17 (0.61)	2797
Relative risks	1.38	1.17(NS)	0.72(NS)	
Caesarean section				
Caesarean section	145 (7.57)	34 (1.78)	12 (0.63)	1915
Vaginal delivery	1372 (14.02)	231 (2.36)	75 (0.77)	9786
Relative risks	1.85	1.33(NS)	1.22(NS)	

TABLE 11.8

Differing durations of stress incontinence, age, birthweight, second stage labour and type of delivery

	Duration 6 weeks – 6 months	Over 6 months	Still persistent	Total women
	No. (%)	No. (%)	No. (%)	
Maternal age				
Up to 24 years	78 (2.97)	43 (1.64)	210 (8.0)	2625
25 – 29 years	130 (3.08)	82 (1.94)	424 (10.04)	4225
30 yrs or more	110 (2.27)	93 (1.92)	610 (12.62)	4851
Relative risks	0.76	1.17(NS)	1.58	
Birthweight				
Up to 3200 grams	109 (2.49)	67 (1.53)	418 (9.54)	4380
3201 – 3700 grams	135 (2.96)	95 (2.08)	467 (10.25)	4557
3701 grams or more	74 (2.68)	56 (2.03)	361 (13.06)	2764
Relative risks	1.08(NS)	1.33	1.37	
Duration of second stage labour (vaginal deliveries only)				
Under 60 mins	175 (2.53)	120 (1.74)	735 (10.64)	6905
60 mins or more	111 (3.97)	78 (2.79)	372 (13.30)	2797
Relative risks	1.57	1.60	1.25	
Caesarean Section				
Caesarean section	29 (1.51)	34 (1.78)	130 (6.79)	1915
Vaginal delivery	289 (2.95)	198 (2.02)	1116 (11.41)	9786
Relative risks	1.91	1.13(NS)	1.68	

Figure 11.2

Urinary Frequency and Associated Factors

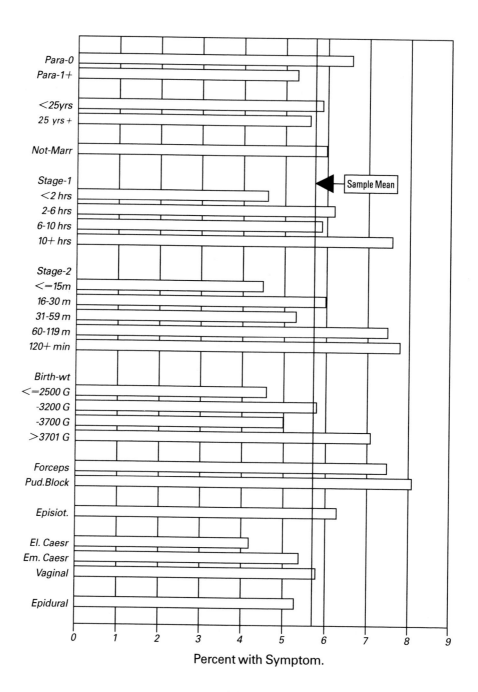

Percent with Symptom.

144

Primary predictors of urinary frequency and secondary associations

Discriminant analyses (Table 11.9) were conducted to separate the primary predictors of urinary frequency from the secondary associations. Only three factors were identified as independent primary predictors: greater birthweight, forceps delivery, and primiparity, the latter exhibiting a relatively weak effect. The analysis of all deliveries, including Caesarean sections, confirmed that Caesarean section was neither a positive nor a negative predictor of this bladder symptom: and that the rates of urinary frequency were the same after emergency and elective sections as after vaginal deliveries (Table 11.9, Column 2).

TABLE 11.9

Discriminant analysis of characteristics associated with urinary frequency

	Vaginal deliveries		All deliveries	
	F value	Coefficients	F value	Coefficients
Heavier Birthweight	9.8780	0.58858	5.888	0.47378
Forceps	8.5810	0.58452	9.8807	0.64225
Primiparity	4.4040	0.42264	4.728	0.44658

Social predictors

The question arose again whether the primiparity relationship with urinary frequency might be an artefact, arising from the selective inclusion of newly occurring symptoms. Subsidiary discriminant analysis of all cases of urinary frequency, new or not, confirmed this supposition. The parity association disappeared.

Obstetric and anaesthetic predictors

Forceps delivery and birthweight

Forceps delivery and increased birthweight were the only independent obstetric predictors of urinary frequency. A separate entry of rotational and straight forceps here had made little difference to the results. In contrast with stress incontinence the discriminant analysis had shown no independent effect of the duration of second stage labour.

Table 11.10 shows the rates of urinary frequency among vaginal deliveries according to parity, birthweight and forceps. The birthweight association was concentrated among primiparae with babies over 3700 grams, and in multiparae who delivered by forceps. The independent effects of forceps were limited to multiparae. There are some similarities between these non-additive findings and those for stress incontinence.

TABLE 11.10

Urinary frequency, parity, birthweight and forceps in vaginal deliveries

	No forceps		Forceps	
		Primiparae		
Birthweight	Urinary frequency No. (%)	Total women	Urinary frequency No. (%)	Total women
Up to 3200 grams	59 (6.5)	901	42 (7.4)	566
3201 – 3700 grams	44 (6.2)	715	35 (5.6)	623
3701 grams or more	22 (8.5)	259	30 (9.1)	331
All weights	125 (6.7)	1875	107 (7.0)	1520
		Multiparae		
Up to 3200 grams	82 (4.4)	1843	15 (7.1)	211
3201 – 3700 grams	106 (4.6)	2298	17 (5.6)	302
3701 grams or more	86 (5.8)	1481	34 (13.3)	256
All weights	274 (4.8)	5662	66 (8.6)	769

Although the length of the second stage was **not** an independent overall predictor of urinary frequency, its relationships with stress incontinence prompted us to look for relationships that might be localised to specific sub-groups. We constructed urinary frequency tabulations according to length of second stage, comparing the use of forceps in primiparae and multiparae separately. There remained no evidence that a longer second stage had any effect, even localised, upon the risk of urinary frequency.

What predicts onset and duration of urinary frequency?

As with stress incontinence, we related the main predictive factors – birthweight and forceps delivery – to different times of onset within and outside the three month period, and to different durations.

Urinary frequency starting in the first post-partum week (82%) was compared with symptoms starting between 2-13 weeks. The associations with both birthweight and forceps were limited to immediate onset symptoms (Table 11.11). Urinary frequency starting more than a week post-delivery was unrelated to delivery factors. Separate discriminant analyses of first-week onsets and of later onsets, confirmed this finding.

TABLE 11.11

Differing onsets of urinary frequency, forceps and birthweight

	Onset Within 1 week No. (%)	2 – 4 weeks No. (%)	5 – 13 weeks No. (%)	3 – 12 months No. (%)	Total women
Forceps	144 (6.26)	17 (0.74)	12 (0.52)	9 (0.39)	2301
No forceps	405 (4.31)	49 (0.52)	41 (0.44)	45 (0.48)	9400
Relative risks	1.43	1.42(NS)	1.18(NS)	0.81(NS)	
Birthweight					
Up to 3700 grams	397 (4.24)	53 (0.59)	40 (0.45)	42 (0.47)	8937
Over 3700 grams	170 (6.15)	13 (0.47)	13 (0.47)	12 (0.43)	2764
Relative risks	1.45	0.80(NS)	1.04(NS)	0.91(NS)	

Urinary frequency still persisting up to the time of questioning was next compared with the more 'transient' symptoms in a similar manner. Most (75%) affected women had reported continuation up to this time. Separate tabulations (Table 11.12) and discriminant analyses showed forceps deliveries and large babies to be equally predictive of urinary frequency of any duration. The restriction of the delivery-factor relationship to early onsets, but its extension to all durations, accords with the findings for stress incontinence.

TABLE 11.12

**Differing durations of urinary frequency,
forceps and birthweight**

	Duration 6 weeks – 6 months No. (%)	Over 6 months No. (%)	Still persistent No. (%)	Total women
Forceps	21 (0.91)	9 (0.39)	134 (5.82)	2301
No forceps	71 (0.76)	24 (0.26)	365 (3.88)	9400
Relative Risks	1.20(NS)	1.50	1.50	
Birthweight				
Up to 3700 grams	62 (0.69)	24 (0.27)	358 (4.01)	8937
Over 3700 grams	30 (1.09)	9 (0.33)	141 (5.10)	2764
Relative Risks	1.58	1.22(NS)	1.27	

Combined bladder symptoms

Of the 668 women with new long-term urinary frequency, 416 also reported new long-term stress incontinence. Combined symptoms amounted to 62.3% of those reporting urinary frequency; but only 23.3% of those reporting stress incontinence. As with backache and headache, the question arose how far the group with combined symptoms resembled those with either symptom alone, and whether any group might differ in its predictors from the others. We conducted separate discriminant analyses for women who had urinary frequency without incontinence (252); or stress incontinence without urinary frequency (1366); or both symptoms (416).

For the combined bladder symptoms, the main independent predictive factors were greater birthweight and forceps delivery, while a Caesarean section delivery had an independent protective effect. Age was not quite significant (F = 3.696). For stress incontinence alone, the positive predictors were a longer second stage, greater birthweight and increasing age, while Caesarean section and Asian ethnic group were negative. For urinary frequency alone, however, these obstetric factors had no relationship at all and primiparity and pudendal block were the only independent predictors. This primiparity association is probably an artefact resulting from the 'first-time' inclusion limitation but the pudendal block effect (although small) could be genuine.

Discussion

One-fifth (20.6%) of all the women in our sample experienced long-term stress incontinence occurring within three months of the delivery; and 15.2% reported it as a new symptom. Most symptoms began immediately, and the majority had not resolved. Even after a first birth, as many as one in ten women experienced newly occurring stress incontinence that had become chronic. Of all the symptoms so far studied, this was the one most specifically related to the delivery of a child.

In the general population the proportion of women with this disorder accumulated over successive deliveries, must be substantial. On the basis of the accurately-dated reports, about 18.9% of women had developed persistent stress incontinence in the course of their first pregnancy and delivery (Table 11.3). Another 15.7% were affected after a second delivery to give a cumulative total of 34.6%, rising through 47% after the third delivery, to 57.6% at the next. From this cumulative total of onsets we should subtract the rather infrequent spontaneous recoveries in order to estimate the cumulated prevalence: although this would probably do little more than balance the incompletely dated – and therefore omitted – cases. The prevalence of stress incontinence in women having had three babies must in the range 40-50%: and among all parous women, about 30-35%.

The apparently falling risk per delivery with increasing parity, as shown in Table 11.3, is deceptive. Allowing for the declining number of those still eligible for a 'first-time' experience of the symptoms, the accumulating rate is close to a constant 19% of those not yet affected, at each successive delivery.

Several studies of stress incontinence in women in the general population have been reported (Thomas 1980; Yarnell et al 1981, 1982; Jolleys 1988), and some found relationships with childbirth events. All found stress incontinence to be a common symptom, more frequent in parous women than in nulliparous women, with the prevalence generally rising with increasing parity. Jolleys (1988), using a general population sample, noted as we have that the full extent of the problem had gone unrecognised because only a small proportion of sufferers consulted their doctors.

Sleep et al. (1984), in a trial of different obstetric perineal management regimes, found that 19% of the women in their sample reported involuntary loss of urine three months after a normal vaginal delivery. This proportion is similar to our own, if we include continuations and recurrences as well as new symptoms. (They did not themselves distinguish these categories).

There are other problems in comparing different estimates, mainly because of difficulties in defining the condition. Stress incontinence has been represented as a continuum, ranging from a slight problem of dampening underwear to one requiring continuous protection against leakage (Jolleys 1988). We were unable in our own study to obtain an assessment of the severity of the recorded symptoms.

Urinary frequency, occurring within three months and persisting more than six weeks was reported by one in ten women, either as a continuation or recurrence of a previous problem, or as a new one: one in twenty women experienced it as a new problem. In almost two thirds of cases, the symptom accompanied stress incontinence, but in the remainder it occurred alone. We could find no published reports on the prevalence or associations of urinary frequency.

The main obstetric predictors of newly occurring stress incontinence, with or without urinary frequency, were prolonged and traumatic deliveries. Caesarean section was 'protective', although not completely so. These predictive factors only applied to those problems which began within about a week of delivery: although they predicted symptoms of lesser and greater duration, equally.

Another important factor for stress incontinence was increasing maternal age. Its association was widely evident among both primiparae and multiparae and following both Caesarean section and vaginal delivery. Jointly with the delivery factors it generated symptom rates ranging from 5.7% in women under 25 years who had a Caesarean section, up to 26.5% in women aged 30 or more who delivered vaginally with a second stage of two hours or more. Unlike the obstetric factors, maternal age were also associated with symptoms starting after the first week. Stress incontinence in older women was also more likely to become chronic. The different onset patterns associated with maternal age and with the delivery factors, the risk of increased age both in vaginal and in non-vaginal deliveries, and the complex relationships with combinations of long labours, forceps and increased birthweight suggest that there may be more than one mechanism in play.

We could not find any reported studies on post-childbirth populations of the effect of maternal age on stress incontinence. The effect of increasing age within childbearing age-groups has been noted in cross-sectional population studies (Yarnell 1981) but this is not exactly equivalent to our own demonstration, which relates to age at childbirth.

Several investigators have commented upon obstetric events affecting the risk of subsequent stress incontinence. Sleep et al (1984; 1986) found no associations between stress incontinence and either episiotomy or laceration. Jolleys (1988) in her general population sample, did find a relationship between perineal sutures and stress incontinence, but no association with the type of delivery. She noted that the small number of abnormal births in the sample rendered the negative results for this last factor, inconclusive. Yarnell (1982) examined the associations of urinary incontinence in an electoral-register-based random sample of 1000 women. There was no association with reports of perineal tear, episiotomy, forceps delivery or Caesarean section, although the authors stated that many women in the sample had experienced them.

Samples based upon general populations present several major difficulties for assessing the role of obstetric factors. The first is the problem of relating the symptoms to events in particular deliveries; the second, is that important details such as the durations of the stages of labour, would not usually be known to the women; the third, is the problem of disentangling the complex inter-relationships between different factors without a full knowledge of all obstetric events and the subsequent application of multivariate analysis. Mainly for such reasons, no doubt, there are no published data-sets comparable with our own, directly relating the types and durations of a particular delivery, or the size of a particular baby, or other maternal factors recorded at the time, to subsequent bladder problems in the mother.

There were some differences of detail in the obstetric predictors of stress incontinence alone, and of stress incontinence combined with urinary frequency. For the combined symptoms, the predominant predictors were forceps delivery and greater birthweight; while for stress incontinence alone these were a longer second stage labour, greater birthweight and increasing age. In both cases Caesarean section was 'protective'. These differences might imply a heterogeneity of etiology, but the details are not easily seen. Some of the contrasts may represent only sampling variations, reflecting the fact that certain of the predictors, such as a long second stage and forceps-usage (as well as the symptom groups) are very closely related.

Urinary frequency alone affected just over 2% of the sample, and was generally unrelated to any of the main social or delivery factors. The only association was with pudendal block, and only eleven women were affected. There could be an entirely different explanation behind this isolated symptom, unconnected with the specific events and procedures of delivery, possibly involving bacterial infection. This must be worthy of further investigation, especially in view of the obvious potential for remedial action.

Snooks et al (1984; 1990) have considered the mechanisms leading to stress incontinence following childbirth. They have proposed that a major factor is damage to the innervation of the pelvic floor musculature, as assessed by electrophysiological techniques. Multiparity, forceps delivery, prolonged second stage labour, third degree tears and high birthweight were all preferentially associated with neural damage. Caesarean section was not associated, indicating that vaginal delivery was a necessary condition for pelvic nerve damage.

Our findings on the predictors of stress incontinence accord in part with those of the above investigators. The results conform with this model in that the most powerful delivery-related predictors of stress incontinence were compatible with high levels of pelvic compressional trauma. Some of our findings however were not compatible. Snooks et al found nerve injury to be commonest in multiparae especially those who were delivered by forceps, and noted that nerve damage after a first birth was occult but reversible. In our data set however chronic symptoms were reported equally after first and subsequent deliveries. In addition Snooks et al (1990) have considered that age – within the range of age at childbirth – was not relevant to innervation damage. But we have shown a quite clear linear association with increasing age, even after Caesarean section, a situation with little opportunity for compressional damage of the intra-pelvic nerves to occur.

This group of previous investigators have focused predominantly upon directly measured nerve damage, while our outcome measures were urinary symptoms as reported by the women. Our findings would be more compatible with a heterogeneous etiology of these post-delivery bladder symptoms.

Chapter 12 – Haemorrhoids

Haemorrhoids, piles, occur during pregnancy and following delivery. Here we were concerned mainly with those presenting as a new problem after the index delivery, so that we could link them with the events recorded in the maternity case notes for a specific delivery.

Frequency of occurrence

Altogether 931 women (8%) reported haemorrhoids beginning for the first time within three months of the index delivery, never experienced before and lasting more than six weeks.

A further 1143 women (9.8%) reported haemorrhoids of similar timing and duration, but which were not new symptoms, bring the total to 18%. Overall there were more recurrent or continuing haemorrhoids than newly occurring; the reverse of the pattern for stress incontinence. In women delivering a first baby however, haemorrhoids were more often a new problem; 60% among primiparae compared with 37% among multiparae. We had not asked about the circumstances of the previous haemorrhoids, but 161 of the 1143 volunteered that they were first experienced after a previous birth, and a further 140 said they had started in the pregnancy and had continued after the birth of the index child. The association between childbirth and haemorrhoids seems to be quite specific, although substantially less than for stress incontinence.

Many additonal women (584) reported haemorrhoids after the index delivery, but did not supply all the items of information necessary for 'acceptance': either the onset date, or the duration, or whether they were recurrent. These inadequately recorded reports were omitted from the following analyses and our investigations were confined to those 931 accurately dated cases where the haemorrhoids had started in the first three months after the delivery, and lasted more than six weeks.

Durations and onsets

Haemorrhoids were rarely transient. Only 16% of the 931 cases had gone within three months, while 70% lasted for more than a year, and 67% were still a problem at the time of our enquiry, thirteen months to nine years later. Many had clearly become chronic.

Although we included as 'affected', all haemorrhoids starting within three months of the delivery, most (85%) of the 931 cases began within the first post-partum week: and 93% within four weeks.

An additional 71 cases of new, long-term haemorrhoids were reported between three and twelve months after the delivery. They were outside our 'acceptance' criteria but the larger total of 1002 first year cases serves to display the temporal specificity of the association with childbirth. Among these 1002 cases, 79% occurred in the first week, and 93% within three months of delivery, again suggesting a close relationship with childbirth.

Medical consultation

The doctor was consulted by 45% of the women reporting haemorrhoids, substantially more than for stress incontinence or for urinary frequency or backache: and about the same as for headache.

As with backache and headache/migraine there was no relationship between the duration or the persistence of the haemorrhoids and the likelihood of consultation, but different types of women were more likely to consult. Affected women in social classes III, IV and V were more likely to visit the doctor (49%) than were affected women in social classes I and II (33%); and 68% of Asian women with reported haemorrhoids had sought medical advice, compared with 44% of Caucasian women.

Most (87%) of the women who consulted with this condition said they were given treatment by their general practitioner, and 6% were referred for specialist consultation and/or treatment. Of the 24 women referred, 17 women said that they had received surgery.

Factors associated with haemorrhoids

The main social factors associated with haemorrhoids are set out in the upper part of Table 12.1 and in Figure 12.1. Primiparous women reported more first-time haemorrhoids than did women having second or later infants. Maternal age at delivery was also associated but the relationship was non-linear, least in women under twenty and over thirty years of age. Tall women had higher rates than short women although there were no significant differences between the social classes in reported frequencies. (Height was also associated with varicose veins. See Chapter 14). Asian women reported much lower rates of haemorrhoids than Caucasians.

The main obstetric associations of haemorrhoids are set out in the lower part of Table 12.1 and in Figure 12.1. Haemorrhoids were more frequent following vaginal delivery than following Caesarean section. They were more often

TABLE 12.1

Characteristics associated with haemorrhoids*

	No. (%)	Total women
Whole sample	931 (8.0)	11701
Parity 0	423 (10.1)	4185
1	386 (8.3)	4669
2+	122 (4.3)	2847
Under 20 years	28 (5.6)	503
20 – 24	179 (8.4)	2122
25 – 29	390 (9.2)	4225
30 or more	334 (6.9)	4851
Married	853 (8.1)	10525
Single/Div/Wid/Sep	78 (6.6) NS	1176
Caucasian	838 (8.3)	10135
Asian	22 (4.2)	530
Height		
Under 155 cms	94 (6.6)	1435
155-159 cms	200 (7.8)	2569
160 cms or more	610 (8.8)	6934
First stage labour		
Under 2 hours	153 (7.4)	2054
2-5 hrs 59 mins	435 (8.3)	5264
6-9 hrs 59 mins	176 (10.5)	1684
10 hours or more	74 (14.5)	511
2nd stage labour		
Up to 5 minutes	20 (3.4)	593
6 – 30 minutes	342 (7.5)	4563
31 – 60 minutes	145 (8.3)	1748
61 – 119 minutes	211 (11.4)	1858
120 – 179 minutes	97 (13.2)	737
180 minutes or more	33 (16.3)	203
Forceps	289 (12.6)	2301
No forceps	642 (6.8)	9400

TABLE 12.1 Cont

Characteristics associated with haemorrhoids*

	No. (%)	Total women
Elective section	24 (3.1)	770
Emergency section	57 (5.0)	1145
Vaginal delivery	850 (8.7)	9786
Episiotomy	528 (10.3)	5112
No episiotomy	403 (6.1)	6589
Pethidine	164 (9.9)	1658
No pethidine	767 (7.6)	10043
General anaesthetic	54 (4.7)	1158
No general anaesthetic	877 (8.3)	10543
Pre-term gestation	46 (5.8)	800
Term gestation	885 (8.1)	10901
Birthweight		
Up to 2500 grams	34 (4.4)	767
2501-3200 grams	271 (7.5)	3613
3201-3700 grams	375 (8.2)	4557
Over 3700 grams	251 (9.1)	2764
Head circumference		
Up to 33 cms	217 (6.9)	3126
34 – 35 cms	484 (8.0)	6044
36 cms or more	223 (9.1)	2459

*Haemorrhoids starting within three months of delivery, never previously experienced, lasting longer than six weeks.

reported after a forceps delivery and after episiotomy, and there was a systematic rise in rates with greater duration of first and second stage labour. Haemorrhoids were more frequent with high infant birthweight and large head circumference, and following delivery at full-term as opposed to pre-term. There was an excess where pethidine was given for pain relief. There was no association with epidural anaesthesia. General anaesthesia was followed by fewer symptoms, probably because of its association with Caesarean section.

Figure 12.1
Haemorrhoids and Associated Factors

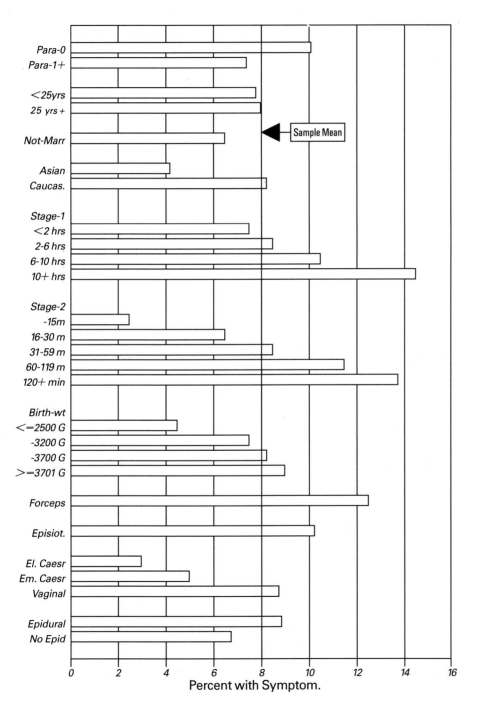

Percent with Symptom.

Primary predictors and secondary associations

Discriminant analysis was undertaken to determine which of these inter-related factors were independently predictive of haemorrhoids. The first column of Table 12.2 shows the results for vaginal deliveries only and includes duration of labour; while the second column related to all delivery types but excludes duration of labour. Primiparity, Caucasian ethnic group and married status were the independent social predictors.

However, the obstetric factors took precedence over the social ones. The independent obstetric predictors included forceps delivery, a longer second stage labour, a heavier baby and (to a lesser extent) the use of pethidine for pain relief. Caesarean section was strongly 'protective'. There were some similarities, here, with stress incontinence.

Social predictors of haemorrhoids

Parity

The reported excess of haemorrhoids in primiparae runs counter to statements in obstetric text books, and the question once more arises whether it is an artefact of the 'recurrence exclusion rule'. When we conducted supplementary

TABLE 12.2

Discriminant analyses of characteristics associated with haemorrhoids

| | Vaginal deliveries | | All deliveries | |
	F-values	Coefficients	F-values	Coefficients
Forceps	12.262	0.38956	32.681	0.48947
Longer 2nd stage labour	10.262	0.38516	N/A	N/A
Heavier birthweight	9.5605	0.29679	13.651	0.29635
Non-Asian ethnic group	7.8459	0.26324	10.525	0.25763
Primiparity	7.4179	0.30523	19.248	0.3906
Married status	7.2081	0.25624	10.100	0.2644
Pethidine	5.2098	0.21733	(3.8348 NS)	
Caesarean section	N/A	N/A	21.480	0.38087
Younger age	NS	NS	4.9332	0.19299

discriminant analysis for all haemorrhoids of the requisite timing and duration, including non-first-time symptoms as well as new occurrences, the association with primiparity disappeared. They were reported by 18.4% of multiparae compared with 16.5% of primiparae. Unlike stress incontinence, haemorrhoids did not show any independent association with maternal age.

Ethnic group

Asian women had only half the rate of haemorrhoids reported by Caucasian women, in marked contrast to the respective proportions seeking medical help. This could stem from language or translation difficulties, leading to problems with the term 'piles' as used in the questionnaire. It probably sometimes took a medical consultation to label piles or haemorrhoids as such. But the difference in prevalence could be real, arising from the considerable variations in dietary patterns.

Marital status

Married women reported higher rates of haemorrhoids and this was significant after taking account of confounding factors including parity, and following the subsidiary discriminant analysis of recurrent, continuing as well as new symptoms. It is difficult to see why this might be.

Obstetric predictors of haemorrhoids

Forceps and duration of second stage labour

A long second stage of labour was closely related to forceps usage: only 6.5% of women with a second stage of up to thirty minutes had forceps, compared with 75% of those lasting two hours or more (see Chapter 6). Unlike stress incontinence, where a prolonged second stage took precedence over forceps as a predictor, both factors remained independently predictive of haemorrhoids. This was true both for first births and for subsequent births.

The separate and combined effects of a long second stage and of forceps delivery are tabulated jointly in Table 12.3. This shows that a longer second stage was associated with higher rates of haemorrhoids both in forceps and non-forceps deliveries; but the additional effect of forceps was present only for second stages lasting an hour or more. With durations under an hour, forceps had no additional effect. This circumscribed picture was equally true in women delivering first and subsequent babies.

TABLE 12.3

Haemorrhoids, forceps and duration of second stage labour among vaginal deliveries

Duration 2nd stage	No forceps		Forceps	
	Haemorrhoids No. (%)	Total women	Haemorrhoids No. (%)	Total women
Up to 15 minutes	192 (6.7)	2881	13 (9.8)	133
16 – 30 minutes	140 (7.2)	1938	17 (8.3)	204
31 – 59 minutes	118 (8.4)	1397	27 (7.7)	351
60 – 89 minutes	61 (8.9)	687	63 (13.9)	452
90 mins – 119 mins	31 (10.3)	302	56 (13.4)	417
120 mins or more	23 (9.4)	245	107 (15.4)	695

Birthweight

Increased birthweight was the third main obstetric predictor of haemorrhoids. We tabulated the association with birthweight after different duration second stages for primiparae and multiparae separately (Table 12.4 and Figure 12.2). This shows that although a longer second stage was associated with higher rates of haemorrhoids for all birthweights, and in both parity groups, greater birthweight had an additional effect only with second stages lasting less than an hour. We conducted the same analysis taking account of forceps, and the same pattern was evident in both forceps and non-forceps deliveries. Increasing birthweight and a longer second stage seemed to act as alternative rather than as additive predictors.

A disproportionate number of low birthweight babies were delivered by Caesarean section. This might account for an apparent birthweight effect. Table 12.5 therefore compares the rates of haemorrhoids at different birthweights among vaginal deliveries only. The effect was still evident and was present among first and among later births. However a similar tabulation of Caesarean sections did not show a birthweight effect; birthweight was relevant only with the vaginal passage of the infant. This resembles the finding for stress incontinence.

TABLE 12.4

Haemorrhoids, birthweight and duration of second stage labour in vaginal deliveries

Duration and birthweight	Primiparae		Multiparae	
	Haemorrhoids No. (%)	Total women	Haemorrhoids No. (%)	Total women
Under 1 hour				
Up to 3200 grams	58 (7.4)	788	99 (5.5)	1804
3201 – 3700 grams	53 (9.9)	533	158 (7.1)	2219
Over 3700 grams	23 (13.5)	170	113 (8.1)	1391
1 hour or more				
Up to 3200 grams	82 (12.2)	673	27 (12.2)	221
3201 – 3700 grams	102 (12.5)	813	34 (9.7)	349
Over 3700 grams	58 (13.8)	420	37 (11.3)	326

Figure 12.2　Haemorrhoids, Birth Wt, Parity & Stage-2

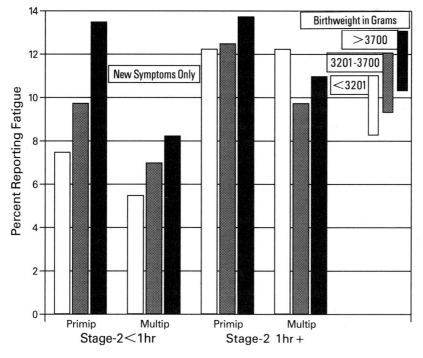

TABLE 12.5

Haemorrhoids, birthweight and parity in vaginal deliveries

| Birthweight | Primiparae | | Multiparae | | All parities | |
	Haemorrhoids No. (%)	Total women	Haemorrhoids No. (%)	Total women	Haemorrhoids No. (%)	Total women
Up to 2500 grams	14 (7.1)	198	9 (3.5)	254	23 (5.1)	452
2501 – 2800 grams	27 (8.5)	316	25 (6.3)	395	52 (7.3)	711
2801 – 3200 grams	102 (10.7)	953	91 (6.5)	1405	193 (8.2)	2358
3201 – 3500 grams	91 (10.6)	855	119 (7.5)	1592	210 (8.6)	2447
3501 – 3700 grams	64 (13.3)	483	77 (7.6)	1008	141 (9.6)	1491
Over 3700 grams	80 (13.6)	590	151 (8.7)	1737	231 (9.9)	2327

Caesarean section

Caesarean section was strongly 'protective' in relation to post-partum haemorrhoids. We looked separately at elective and emergency Caesarean sections, since most of the latter also have a period in labour, and this might be relevant (Table 12.6). The first crude comparisons had shown higher rates after an emergency section (Table 12.1 and Figure 12.1) but after taking account of parity, since primiparae have more emergency sections, this difference disappeared.

TABLE 12.6

Haemorrhoids, type of delivery and parity		
	Haemorrhoids No. (%)	Total women
Primiparae		
Elective section	6 (3.8)	158
Emergency section	39 (6.2)	632
Vaginal delivery	378 (11.1)	3395
Multiparae		
Elective section	18 (2.9)	612
Emergency section	18 (3.5)	513
Vaginal delivery	472 (7.4)	6391

Pethidine

There was an independent association between haemorrhoids and the use of pethidine for pain relief. It is difficult to explain. It was not due to an association between pethidine and long labour, because detailed tabulations showed that the excess of haemorrhoids associated with pethidine was restricted to women experiencing a shorter second stage.

163

What predicts onsets and durations of haemorrhoids?

The main analyses related to first-time haemorrhoids, starting within three months of delivery and lasting more than six weeks, but we also examined onsets and durations, within and outside these limits.

The onset analysis was the most informative. All the main predictors of haemorrhoids were associated exclusively with those symptoms which started within a week of delivery (Table 12.7). Onsets between two and thirteen weeks after the birth, were as unrelated to these predictors as were haemohoids which first appeared after 3 months. This was the same as for stress incontinence and for urinary frequency. Subsidiary discriminant analyses of haemorrhoids starting in the first week and of those starting in weeks 2 to 13, confirmed these findings.

TABLE 12.7

Differing onsets of haemorrhoids and main predictors

	Onset Within 1 week	2 – 4 weeks	5 – 13 weeks	3 – 12 months	Total women
Second stage*					
Under 1 hour	424 (6.14)	47 (0.68)	37 (0.54)	41 (0.59)	6905
1 hour or more	300 (10.73)	21 (0.75)	19 (0.68)	19 (0.68)	2797
Relative Risks	1.75	1.10 (NS)	1.26 (NS)	1.15 (NS)	
Forceps*	258 (11.21)	16 (0.70)	15 (0.66)	16 (0.70)	2301
No forceps	469 (6.27)	51 (0.68)	41 (0.55)	44 (0.59)	7485
Relative Risks	1.79	1.03 (NS)	1.20 (NS)	1.19 (NS)	
Birthweight					
Up to 3700 grams	567 (6.34)	59 (0.66)	54 (0.60)	45 (0.50)	8937
More than 3700 grams	224 (8.10)	14 (0.51)	13 (0.47)	26 (0.94)	2764
Relative Risks	1.28	0.83 (NS)	0.78 (NS)	1.88	
Section	64 (3.34)	17 (0.89)		12 (0.63)	1915
No section	727 (7.43)	123 (1.26)		60 (0.61)	9786
Relative Risks	2.22	1.42 (NS)		0.97 (NS)	

*Vaginal deliveries only

TABLE 12.8

Differing durations of haemorrhoids and main predictors

	Duration 6 weeks- 3 months	3 – 6 months	6 – 12 months	Over 12 months	Still persistent	Total
Second stage*	78 (1.13)	47 (0.68)	28 (0.41)	22 (0.32)	333 (4.82)	6905
1 hour or more	47 (1.68)	36 (1.29)	17 (0.61)	12 (0.42)	228 (8.15)	2797
Relative Risks	1.49	1.90	1.49	1.31 (NS)	1.69	
Forceps*	42 (1.83)	28 (1.22)	14 (0.61)	11 (0.48)	194 (8.48)	2301
No forceps	84 (1.12)	55 (0.73)	31 (0.41)	22 (0.29)	369 (4.92)	7485
Relative Risks	1.63	1.67	1.49	1.66	1.72	
Birthweight						
Up to 3700 gramms	89 (1.0)	72 (0.81)	37 (0.41)	28 (0.31)	456 (5.10)	8937
More than 3700 grams	46 (1.66)	20 (0.72)	12 (0.43)	8 (0.29)	165 (5.97)	2764
Relative Risks	1.66	0.89 (NS)	1.05 (NS)	0.94 (NS)	1.17 (NS)	
Section	9 (0.47)	9 (0.47)	4	1	58 (3.03)	1915
No section	126 (1.29)	83 (0.85)	45	33	563 (5.75)	9786
Relative Risks	2.74	1.81	3.08		1.90	

*Vaginal deliveries only

On the other hand, symptoms of all durations over six weeks were predicted equally by each of the main factors (Table 12.8). Forceps delivery, a long second stage labour and a heavier baby were as predictive of shorter symptoms lasting six weeks to three months, as of those still present at the time of our enquiry: and Caesarean section was equally 'protective.'

Discussion

Haemorrhoids occurring after childbirth are a problem familiar to practising midwives and obstetricians. They have been said to result from the action of progesterone on the bowel, from constipation during pregnancy, and from pelvic pressure causing increased varicosity. Obstetric textbooks generally note that they can cause a great deal of pain for the first few days of the puerperium; they are then said usually to disappear, although they are more likely to become worse with each successive pregnancy, and can become permanent. (Hibbard 1988; Iffy and Kaminetzky 1981; Knor 1987) Apart from such references to the effect of increasing parity, we found no investigations in the literature on any of the social or obstetric factors which predisposed to haemorrhoids: nor has the prevalence been measured, or their extension beyond the immediate post-partum period been adequately documented.

In this population newly occurring haemorrhoids, lasting for longer than six weeks, developed after one delivery in twelve: persistence was common, such that one in twenty women in our population still complained of haemorrhoids at the time of questioning, thirteen months to nine years after the birth. The frequency of new occurrences was even higher after a first baby, where one in ten developed long-term piles and one in fourteen reported their persistence.

Haemorrhoids of early post-partum onset were clearly related to pelvic trauma. They were much more likely after long second stage labours, forceps deliveries and the vaginal delivery of larger infants. Caesarean section was protective and, here, birthweight had no effect. The variation produced by these combined predictors was considerable. Following Caesarean section only 4.2% of women reported subsequent haemorrhoids, compared with 18% after a forceps delivery following a second stage of three hours or more. Symptoms which appeared after the first week however showed no relationship with any of these delivery factors. This finding reflected the pattern seen with stress incontinence and urinary frequency.

Asian women reported haemorrhoids less often, but a higher proportion of those who did had attended their doctor, suggesting that an 'assisted-diagnosis' might be required before these women would report. However, given the considerable differences in Asian and Caucasian diets these reduced rates could be real. Our study was directly concerned only with childbirth factors, but this suggests that inappropriate diets might first predispose some women towards the condition.

Even though we specifically refer to haemorrhoids as new symptoms, first appearing after delivery, and usually immediately, symptom initiation might have begun during the pregnancy, or even before. It might sometimes be that the trauma of a long or a forceps delivery or a large baby then worsens the condition, with the haemorrhoids becoming thrombosed or prolapsed, and consequently symptomatic and obvious to the woman.

Some women are probably more susceptible than others, some for reasons irrespective of childbirth, and some as a result of it. The ethnic differences, and the data relating to parity variations provide evidence of this. Our results indicate that the risk of new haemorrhoids is greater after a first birth, and when measured in relation to women thus far unaffected, it declines with each successive birth. This differs from stress incontinence, where the risk of new symptoms among unaffected women remained nearly constant. Allowing for reductions in the numbers of women surviving as eligibles for new symptoms, the rate for new haemorrhoids after first and subsequent births were approximately 10.1%, 9.2% and 6%. Once they had appeared, however, all of them were equally long-lasting. Reassurances in obstetric text-books that haemorrhoids usually become permanent only after several deliveries, are misplaced.

Chapter 13 – Depression, Anxiety and Extreme Tiredness

The women were asked in the questionnaire whether they had experienced depression or anxiety since having their baby. Depression and anxiety are generally regarded as distinct clinical diagnoses, but the component symptoms can overlap. It was not practical to try to separate them using a limited postal questionnaire, while pursuing our broad objectives. The responses do not therefore represent a homogeneous diagnostic group, but rather a group of women with a range of post-partum mental health problems which either they or their doctors regarded as depression or anxiety.

We also asked about 'extreme tiredness'. Fatigue after giving birth is commonly regarded as normal and not strictly a 'health problem', but depending on its duration and severity, it might still be disabling. For this reason, and because we could find no previous investigations of the topic, we decided to include it. Self-reporting of extreme tiredness, more than most complaints, will be affected by individual expectations and perceptions: what one woman regards as disabling and reportable might be regarded by another as normal and unworthy of report. Within our restricted questionnaire we had to rely on the women's own interpretations.

Our purpose in enquiring into these symptoms sprang from a primary interest in their frequencies and in their origins; but we were also concerned whether women with post-partum mental ill-health might differ in their perceptions of other health problems such as backache or headache or incontinence, and report them excessively. If mood disturbance followed from particular circumstances or procedures (e.g. an induction or general anaesthesia) or if longstanding mood disturbances had precipitated the use of other procedures (e.g. epidurals), then results relating to all symptoms could be seriously biased. We needed to take precautions against these possibilities, and this was a secondary reason for asking these questions.

Frequency of occurrence

Altogether a total of 1065 women, 9.1% of the sample, reported 'anxiety or depression' which they had not experienced before, commencing within three months of the index delivery and lasting more than six weeks. As with other symptoms, our main analyses were limited to this group. However, an additional 498 women (4.3%) reported anxiety/depression of like onset and duration, but which was not a new symptom. The total, of new occurrences together with continuing or recurrent problems, amounted to 13.4% of the population.

Despite the self perception problems, and the consequent difficulties of interpretation, there was clear evidence of childbirth-specificity. The majority of affected women (68%) said they were experiencing depression/anxiety for the first time, and among primiparae this was 77% against 61% among multiparae. On this evidence a large number of all episodes were thus associated with childbirth, either the 'index' delivery or a previous one.

A further 360 women reported depresssion some time after the index delivery, but did not give all the details necessary for 'acceptance' into our main analyses. Our estimates of prevalence must therefore be regarded as minima.

A total of 1427 women (12.2%) reported 'extreme tiredness', starting within three months of the birth, persisting for more than six weeks, and not experienced in that form before. As with anxiety/depression, and for similar reasons, it was this group on which we based our main analyses. However, an additional 572 women (4.9%) reported the same form of complaint, except that they had also experienced it before. Like depression, the majority of complaints (71%) were new: and among primiparae 82%, compared with 63% of those having a second or later child. As with depression/anxiety this suggests a high level of childbirth-specificity.

Many additional women (522) reported extreme tiredness after the index delivery, but did not give all the information necessary for inclusion. As with depression/anxiety these cases were omitted from the analyses, but again indicate that our estimates of prevalence are to be regarded as low.

Extreme fatigue is a recognised symptom of depression/anxiety, and not surprisingly, we found a cross-association between the two symptoms. There were 496 women (from among the 1065 with depression and the 1427 with extreme tiredness) who reported both symptoms: almost half (47%) of the women with depression and a third (35%) of those with fatigue. There were 596 women reporting depression without tiredness, and 931 who reported tiredness but not depression.

For our main analyses we concentrate first upon the 1065 women with newly occurring and adequately specified depression/anxiety, with or without fatigue,; then the 1427 women with extreme tiredness, with or without depression/anxiety. Finally, we examine the group of 496 women who reported both conditions, and we compare the separate groups.

Durations and onsets

'Depression' was shorter lived than most of the other post-partum health problems; 18% of the 1065 affected women reported durations of only six weeks to three months; and 60% had resolved within a year. Only 27% of the women with depression said they still had it at the time of our enquiry.

Extreme tiredness lasted longer but was still less persistent than the problems described in previous chapters. In 14% of the 1427 cases it lasted six weeks to three months, and in 50% had resolved within a year. Only 39% of the affected women still complained of extreme fatigue at the time of questioning. Women with combined symptoms had durations similar to those with extreme tiredness.

Most of the 1427 women with extreme fatigue (73%) reported onsets in the first post-partum week: and 89% had started within the first four weeks. For depression the onsets were more widely spread over the first three post-partum months, with 55% of the 1065 reported onsets within a week of the delivery, 78% within four weeks. This pattern of onset accords with the literature on this topic.

Although excluded from our main analyses, we noted all new long-term symptoms beginning in the remainder of the first post-partum year. An additional 221 women reported new depression starting three to twelve months after the delivery and 178 reported extreme tiredness. This makes a total of 1286 new cases of depression within the first year, and 1605 of tiredness. Among all these depressions, 46% began within a week of the delivery, 65% within four weeks and 83% within three months. With extreme tiredness, 65% started within a week of delivery, 79% within four weeks and 89% within three months. This confirms the high level of childbirth-specificity already noted on other grounds.

Medical consultation

Consultation rates with general practitioners for depression were relatively high; 48% (514) of the affected women had consulted. The likelihood of attendance was linked with the duration of the condition, which might therefore be regarded as a marker of severity. For depressions lasting six weeks to three months, 31% of the women consulted; compared with 46% of those lasting three months to a year, and 59% of those lasting more than a year. More than half of those consulting (52%) were given tablets, 8% reported other forms of treatment, mostly relaxation therapy or counselling, and only 11% of those consulting said they were referred for specialist advice or treatment.

Medical consultation rates for extreme tiredness were lower; only 26% said they had consulted a doctor. Reporting an illness as 'depression' or as 'extreme tiredness' may in some cases have depended as much upon the circumstances leading to its labelling as upon the nature of the condition: and this in turn upon whether the women sought medical advice. Again, a positive relationship existed between the duration of fatigue and the consultation rate: only 13% of women with extreme tiredness lasting six weeks to three months went to the doctor, compared with 34% where it lasted longer than a year.

Women who reported both depression and tiredness, consulted a doctor more frequently than those with tiredness alone, but less frequently than those with depression alone. Double reporting does not seem here, to be an indicator of severity or of concern.

The frequency of medical consultations differed according to ethnic group but in opposite directions for the two symptoms. Asian women reporting extreme fatigue more frequently consulted the doctor (45%) than did Caucasian women (26%). But those reporting depression were less likely to consult: 39% compared with 49% of symptomatic Caucasians. Maternal age, marital status and social class were not related to the likelihood of medical consultation for either condition, but there was a small parity difference for extreme tiredness: 23% of affected women attended after a first baby and 29% following a subsequent birth.

Factors associated with depression

The chief associations of anxiety/depression are shown in Table 13.1 and in Figure 13.1, with the social factors set out in the upper part. Primiparous women reported higher rates of depression, as did younger women, and women who were single, divorced, separated or widowed, compared with those who were married.

The main obstetric associations of depression are set out in the lower part of Table 13.1. The variations in rates were moderate but they were widely distributed and not specifically associated with any particular obstetric events and circumstances. This was in contrast to the spinal axis and the pelvic symptoms described in earlier chapters. There were small excesses in women with abnormal fetal presentations, with epidurals, with general anaesthesia and with pudendal block. There were gradients according to the durations of first and second stages of labour and a concordant small excess with forceps. Caesarean sections, post-partum haemorrhage and low infant birthweights were also associated with a modest increase in the rates of depression.

TABLE 13.1

**Characteristics associated with depression/anxiety
and extreme tiredness***

	Depression/anxiety		Extreme tiredness		Total
	No.	(%)	No.	(%)	women
Whole sample	1065	(9.1)	1427	(12.2)	11701
Parity 0	507	(12.1)	680	(16.2)	4185
1	375	(8.0)	489	(10.5)	4669
2+	183	(6.4)	258	(9.1)	2847
Under 25 years	291	(11.1)	289	(11.0)	2625
25 – 34	669	(8.7)	936	(12.2)	7688
35 or more	105	(7.6)	202	(14.6)	1388
Married	917	(8.7)	1255	(11.9)	10525
Single/Div/Sep/Wid	148	(12.6)	172	(14.6)	1176
Social Class					
I and II	258	(8.9) NS	409	(14.2)	2882
III, IV & V	603	(8.6)	812	(11.5)	7048
Singleton	1043	(9.0)	1393	(12.1)	11532
Multiple	22	(13.0)	34	(20.1)	169
Occipito-Anterior	904	(8.8)	1224	(11.9)	10265
Other presentations	161	(11.3)	202	(14.1)	1430
First stage labour					
Under 2 hours	141	(6.9)	206	(10.0)	2054
2 – 5 hrs 59 mins	446	(8.5)	624	(11.9)	5264
6 – 9 hrs 59 mins	183	(10.9)	229	(13.6)	1684
10 hours or more	67	(13.1)	90	(17.6)	511
Second stage labour					
Up to 15 minutes	230	(7.6)	301	(10.1)	3014
16 – 30 minutes	170	(7.9)	234	(10.9)	2142
31 – 59 minutes	164	(9.4)	222	(12.7)	1748
60 – 119 minutes	178	(9.6)	253	(13.6)	1858
120 minutes or more	112	(11.9)	155	(16.5)	940
Rotational forceps	50	(11.3)	77	(17.4)	443
Straight forceps	187	(10.1)	244	(13.1)	1858
No forceps	828	(8.8)	1106	(11.8)	9400

TABLE 13.1 Cont.

	Depression/anxiety No. (%)	Extreme tiredness No. (%)	Total women
Elective section	79 (10.3)	90 (11.7)	770
Emergency section	133 (11.6)	170 (14.8)	1145
Vaginal delivery	853 (8.7)	1167 (11.9)	9785
Episiotomy	480 (9.4) NS	665 (13.0)	5112
No episiotomy	585 (8.9)	762 (11.6)	6589
Post-partum haemorrhage	164 (11.0)	244 (16.4)	1487
No PPH	901 (8.8)	1183 (11.6)	10214
Epidural	478 (10.0)	617 (12.9)	4766
No epidural	587 (8.5)	810 (11.7)	6935
General anaesthesia	131 (11.3)	150 (13.0) NS	1158
No general anaesthesia	934 (8.9)	1277 (12.1)	10543
Pethedine	169 (10.2) NS	230 (13.9)	1658
No pethedine	896 (8.6)	1197 (11.9)	10043
Inhalation	426 (8.7) NS	647 (13.2)	4916
No inhalation	639 (9.4)	780 (11.5)	6785
Pudendal block	37 (13.0)	36 (12.7) NS	284
No pudendal block	1028 (9.0)	1391 (12.2)	11417
Birthweight			
Up to 2500 grams	75 (9.8)	98 (12.8)	767
2501-3200 grams	368 (10.2)	453 (12.5)	3613
3201-3700 grams	393 (8.6)	553 (12.1)	4557
3701 grams or more	229 (8.3)	823 (11.7)	2764
Breast feeding	749 (9.4) NS	1052 (13.3)	7937
Artificial feeding	316 (8.4)	375 (10.0)	3764

*Complaints starting within three months of delivery, never previously experienced, lasting longer than six weeks.

Figure 13.1

Depression and Associated Factors

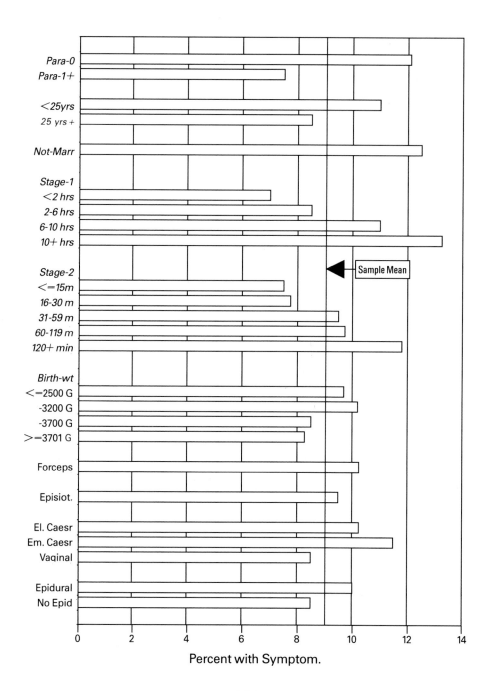

Percent with Symptom.

Primary predictors of depression and secondary associations

Discriminant analysis identified the independent predictors of depression, after taking all the others into account. The two standard sets of results are displayed in Table 13.2, for vaginal deliveries, and for all delivery types. The significant primary predictors of depression were primiparity, a longer first stage labour, non-married status, multiple pregnancy, breast feeding, low infant birthweight and Caesarean section. We examined them further.

Social predictors

Parity and age

Some previous investigators have found postnatal depression to be more frequent among primiparae, but others have found the reverse. Interpretation of our own parity and age relationships was again problematical because of the exclusion of recurrent or continuing complaints. When we repeated the discriminant analyses for all depressions 'first time' or recurrent, the primiparity effect was diminished, but it remained statistically significant. Maternal age remained non-significant overall.

Looking for any localised effects within specific age and parity sub-groups, we tabulated depression according to age among primiparae and multiparae separately (Table 13.3). This showed (Column 1) an excess among younger multiparae, but not among younger primiparae. Separate subsidiary discriminant analyses among primiparae and multiparae separately, confirmed this relationship. Table 13.3 (Column 2) also tabulates new and recurrent depressions together. Among primiparae an excess among older women became evident. The interpretation of these complex relationships becomes clear later, in the combined depression and fatigue analyses.

Marital status

Women recorded as not married in the maternity case-notes had more depression, even after taking related factors into account (Table 13.2). 'Unmarried' included single, divorced, separated or widowed, and there were no differences in rates between these separate groups. Some of the unmarried women would have been living with the baby's father as if married (although we have no data on the proportion), but others would be subject to the social, economic and environmental pressures of living alone, which could lead to stress and depression.

TABLE 13.2

Discriminant analysis of characteristics associated with depression

	Vaginal deliveries		All deliveries	
	F value	Co-efficient	F value	Co-efficient
Primiparity	16.023	0.45693	59.098	0.82426
Longer 1st stage labour	13.221	0.40135	N/A	N/A
Unmarried status	11.760	0.36668	9.6906	0.33418
Multiple pregnancy	7.5241	0.29363	NS	NS
Section	N/A	N/A	8.7495	0.3136
Breast feeding	4.6627	0.22863	NS	NS
Lower birthweight	3.9050	0.21482	NS	NS

TABLE 13.3

Depression, age and parity

	Depression No. (%)	Depression, including recurrences No. (%)	Total women
Primiparae			
Under 25 years	194 (12.5)	245 (15.7)	1558
25 – 29 years	170 (11.1)	215 (14.1)	1527
30 years or more	143 (13.0)	196 (17.8)	1100
All ages	507 (12.1)	656 (15.7)	4185
Multiparae			
Under 25 years	97 (9.1)	140 (13.1)	1067
25 – 29 years	209 (7.7)	331 (12.3)	2698
30 years or more	252 (6.7)	436 (11.6)	3751
All ages	558 (7.4)	907 (12.1)	7516

Information on marital status is collected at the first hospital antenatal visit, usually early in pregnancy and some women marry between then and the birth. Marriage is more likely during a first pregnancy, so that a greater proportion of the primiparae categorised as 'unmarried' would have been married by the time of the birth. We compared the proportions of married and unmarried women reporting depression among first births and subsequent births. (Table 13.4). The unmarried excess was significant only among the multiparae although the association among the primiparae was in the same direction.

TABLE 13.4

Depression, marital status and parity

	Depression, No. (%)	Total women
Married primiparae	410 (11.8)	3483
Unmarried primiparae	97 (13.8)	702
Married multiparae	507 (7.2)	7042
Unmarried multiparae	51 (10.8)	474

Breast feeding

Discriminant analysis showed that breast feeding at the time of hospital discharge was an independent predictor of subsequent depression (Table 13.2), although a weak one. It had not shown up as a simple association (Table 13.1). The constant ties entailed in breast feeding and the additional fatigue arising from the inability to share feeding responsibilities might explain it. Unfortunately the data available on infant feeding were not satisfactory: we knew only the feeding style at the time of hospital discharge and a high proportion of mothers who initially breast feed are known to stop soon after.

Obstetric predictors

Duration of first stage labour

Table 13.1 showed simple correlations of symptoms with longer first and second stages of labour. The two durations were themselves closely related, but under discriminant analysis the duration of the first stage took precedence. This is the reverse of the findings for backache, stress incontinence and haemorrhoids. We compared rates of depression according to the length of the first stage in primiparae and multiparae separately, and the association was equally strong in each.

One problem in interpreting any association with the duration of the first stage is its dependence upon the woman's own perception of the time of 'onset', usually before admission to hospital. Some women would associate the onset of labour with levels of uterine contraction that would be disregarded by other women. There could be a correlation between the precursors of depression and a tendency to report an early onset labour.

Multiple pregnancy

The observed association between depression and twins or triplets could be due to the extra stresses and fatique involved in caring for more than one baby. Among the 169 women with a multiple birth, the crude relative risk of depression was 1.44. It remained significant after taking account of inter-related factors, although its numerical contribution to the occurrence of postnatal depression is small.

Caesarean section

Caesarean section was positively and independently predictive of subsequent depression. Some previous studies have reported the same. This is the reverse of the pelvic trauma associations of bladder symptoms and haemorrhoids. We examined this further comparing both types of section, and the different type of anaesthesia used; and because elective sections are less common among women delivering a first baby, we examined the associations separately according to parity.

We found that the excess of depression after a section seemed to be confined to women delivering a first baby (Table 13.5). There was no significant difference

TABLE 13.5

Depression, parity and Caesarean section

	Primiparae		Multiparae	
	Depression	Total	Depression	Total
	No. %	women	No. %	women
Section	114 (14.4)	790	98 (8.7)	1125
Vaginal	393 (11.6)	3395	460 (7.6)	6391

between the different types of section; and the type of anaesthesia used made no difference either.

Among multiparae the lack of an apparent association with Caesarean section might have been masked by the exclusion of all recurrent symptoms. More multiparae delivering by section would have had previous sections; and if the first section was associated with depression then a higher proportion of women with second sections would be excluded. We therefore re-examined this among multiparae including both new and recurrences of depression, but still there was no association with Caesarean section. The relationship did indeed seem limited to first births.

Birthweight

There was more depression after the delivery of smaller babies. As with Caesarean section, this is the opposite of the pelvic trauma associations of bladder problems and haemorrhoids. Small infants are more frequently delivered by Caesarean section and more common among first births, both factors already shown to be predictors of depression. This might account for the birthweight association. The lack of a significant association for birthweight in the discriminant analysis that included Caesarean deliveries (Table 13.2, Column 2) seemed to support the suggestion that the birthweight effect occurred via the Caesarean effect. However a tabulation of depression according to birthweight and type of delivery, among primiparae and multiparae separately, showed that the birthweight association was not an artefact. There are indeed plausible mechanisms through which a small baby could cause stress, including extra concern as to its well-being; difficulty over feeding; and more frequent waking. The relationship with birthweight however was relatively weak, and it does seem likely from this evidence that it could play a major part in the etiology of post-partum depression.

179

What predicts onsets and durations of depression?

The main analyses of symptoms relate to first-time depressions starting within three months of delivery and lasting longer than six weeks. However we carried out additional tabulations and discriminant analyses for different times and different durations within and outside these limits.

There were some differences in the main predictors according to times of onset but they were not as striking as for the bladder symptoms and for haemorrhoids (Table 13.6). The main features were that depression following a Caesarean section seemed to be limited to depression starting after the first post-delivery week, while the long labour association was present for all onsets up to four weeks but not afterwards. The onset of depression associated with twins tended to be immediate. The depressions starting three to twelve months after delivery, (excluded from our 'affected' group) were not associated with any of the predictive factors (Table 13.5). All these onset associations were confirmed as being independent ones in separate discriminant analyses of the immediate and the later onset symptoms.

Table 13.7 shows similar breakdowns for depression according to the different durations. Primiparity and a long first stage predicted the full range of symptom durations, but unmarried status and multiple pregnancy were especially associated with depressions that had still not been resolved at the time of our enquiry. These findings were confirmed by separate discriminant analyses of depressions with different durations.

Factors associated with extreme tiredness

The simple social and demographic statistical associations of extreme tiredness are shown in the upper part of Table 13.1 and in Figure 13.2. As with depression, primiparous women, unmarried women and women who were breast feeding all reported higher rates. Unlike depression, fatigue was reported more by older women. This association with increasing maternal age was in a direction opposite to that indicated by the primiparity relationship.

Many different obstetric and anaesthetic factors exhibited simple statistical associations with extreme tiredness, as shown in the lower part of Table 13.1. Again, like depression, the associations were widely distributed and not obviously focused upon particular events or procedures. Women with multiple pregnancies and atypical fetal presentations reported higher rates, as did those with longer first and second stages of labour. Epidural anaesthesia, pethidine, inhalation analgesia, episiotomy, forceps delivery, emergency Caesarean section and post-partum haemorrhage were all associated with more fatigue.

TABLE 13.6

Differing onsets of depression and main predictors

	Onset Within 1 week No. (%)	2 – 4 weeks No. (%)	5 – 13 weeks No. (%)	3 – 12 months No. (%)	Total women
Parity					
Primiparae	299 (7.14)	106 (2.53)	102 (2.44)	80 (1.91)	4185
Multiparae	288 (3.83)	138 (1.84)	132 (1.76)	141 (1.87)	7516
Relative risks	1.86	1.38	1.39	1.02 (NS)	
Marital status					
Married	502 (4.77)	215 (2.04)	200 (1.90)	192 (1.82)	10525
Unmarried	85 (7.23)	29 (2.47)	34 (2.89)	29 (2.47)	1176
Relative risks	1.52	1.21 (NS)	1.52	1.36 (NS)	
Multiple pregnancy					
Multiple	14 (8.28)	8 (4.73)		3 (1.78)	169
Singleton	573 (4.97)	470 (4.08)		218 (1.89)	11532
Relative risks	1.67	1.16 (NS)		0.94 (NS)	
Duration					
First Stage labour					
Under six hours	313 (4.28)	133 (1.82)	141 (1.93)	127 (1.74)	7318
Six hours or more	148 (6.74)	57 (2.60)	45 (2.05)	46 (2.10)	2195
Relative risks	1.57	1.43	1.06 (NS)	1.21 (NS)	
Caesarean section					
Section	111 (5.80)	52 (2.72)	49 (2.56)	41 (2.14)	1915
Vaginal	476 (4.86)	192 (1.96)	185 (1.89)	180 (1.84)	9786
Relative risks	1.19 (NS)	1.39	1.35	1.16 (NS)	

TABLE 13.7

Differing durations of depression and main predictors

	Duration 6 weeks-3 months No. (%)	3 – 6 months No. (%)	6 – 12 months No. (%)	Over 12 months No. (%)	Still persistent No. (%)	Total women
Parity						
Primiparae	73 (1.74)	120 (2.87)	122 (2.92)	59 (1.41)	133 (3.18)	4185
Multiparae	78 (1.04)	127 (1.69)	115 (1.53)	79 (1.05)	159 (2.12)	7516
Relative risks	1.69	1.70	1.91	1.30	1.50	
Marital status						
Not married	17 (1.44)	22 (1.87)	29 (2.47)	16 (1.36)	64 (5.44)	1176
Married	134 (1.27)	225 (2.14)	208 (1.98)	122 (1.16)	228 (2.17)	10525
Relative risks	1.13(NS)	1.14(NS)	1.25(NS)	1.17(NS)	2.51	
Multiple pregnancy						
Multiple	7* (4.14)			7 (4.14)	8 (4.73)	169
Singleton	628 (5.44)			131 (1.14)	284 (2.46)	11532
Relative risks	0.76(NS)			3.63	1.92	
Duration 1st stage labour						
Under 6 hours	83 (1.13)	135 (1.84)	133 (1.82)	77 (1.05)	159 (2.17)	7318
6 hours or more	37 (1.69)	59 (2.69)	47 (2.14)	34 (1.55)	73 (3.33)	2195
Relative risks	1.50	1.46	1.18(NS)	1.48	1.53	
Caesarean section						
Section	28 (1.46)	51 (2.66)	50 (2.61)	31 (1.62)	52 (2.72)	1915
Vaginal	123 (1.26)	196 (2.0)	187 (1.91)	107 (1.09)	240 (2.45)	9786
Relative risks	1.16(NS)	1.33	1.37	1.49	1.11(NS)	

*The includes all durations up to 12 months

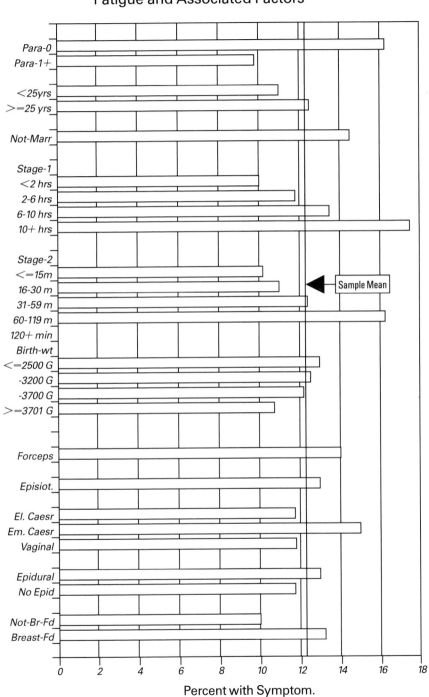

Figure 13.2
Fatigue and Associated Factors

Sample Mean

Percent with Symptom.

Primary predictors of extreme tiredness and secondary associations

Discriminant analysis, undertaken to disentangle primary independent associations from those more likely to be secondary, showed that all the social factors identified above had independent effects (Table 13.8). The two main ones were primiparity and increased maternal age. Post-partum haemorrhage, the use of inhalation analgesia, multiple pregnancy and a longer first stage of labour, were the main obstetric predictors. There were similarities here with depression, although Caesarean section was not implicated.

TABLE 13.8

Discriminant analyses of characteristics associated with extreme tiredness

| | Vaginal deliveries | | All deliveries | |
	F-values	Coefficients	F-values	Coefficients
Primiparity	68.651	0.72727	107.29	0.75348
Older age	29.502	0.47249	38.891	0.47597
Inhalation	12.250	0.27518	16.937	0.28499
Breast feeding	9.8665	0.25012	9.581	0.21796
Post-partum haemorrhage	8.9378	0.23608	20.730	0.31548
Longer 1st stage labour	8.1288	0.23487	N/A	N/A
Multiple pregnancy	8.0747	0.22289	9.3095	0.20896
Unmarried status	5.033	0.19373	11.591	0.24573
Social class I & II	NS	NS	7.7531	0.19937

Social predictors

Parity and age

The positive association between primiparity and extreme fatigue might have resulted from the exclusion of recurrent symptoms; but the maternal age association was in the opposite direction. Additional discriminant analyses, including recurrent and continuing as well as new cases of long-term fatigue, confirmed the predictive pre-eminence of primiparity and of increased age at maternity. Neither could be explained in terms of the other or as selective artefacts. They remained real and powerful predictors.

We sub-tabulated the relationship between age and first-time reports among primiparae and multiparae separately, shown in Table 13.9 and in Figure 13.3. The increased rates of first-time fatigue with increasing age were clear in both parity groups, and the primiparity effect was evident at all ages. The highest rates of all were in women who had delivered a first baby at age thirty years or more, when one in five reported this complaint. We might have anticipated that older women with more than one child to care for would have most tiredness, but this was not the case. Table 13.8 also shows the numbers of women

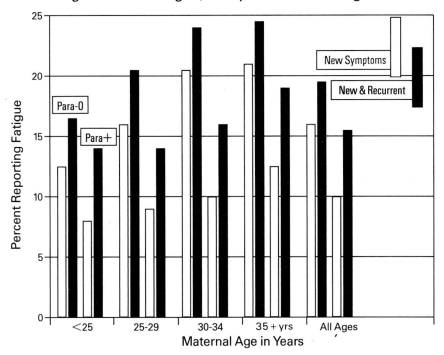

Figure 13.3 Fatigue, Parity and Maternal Age

TABLE 13.9

Extreme tiredness, parity and maternal age

Maternal age	Primiparae Extreme tiredness No. (%)	Primiparae Extreme tiredness including recurrences No. (%)	Total women	Multiparae Extreme tiredness No. (%)	Multiparae Extreme tiredness including recurrences No. (%)	Total women
Under 25 yrs	197 (12.6)	255 (16.4)	1558	92 (8.6)	151 (14.2)	1067
25 – 29 years	257 (16.8)	310 (20.3)	1527	250 (9.3)	384 (14.2)	2698
30 – 34 years	164 (20.3)	193 (23.8)	810	265 (10.0)	434 (16.4)	2653
35 yrs or more	62 (21.4)	72 (24.8)	290	140 (12.8)	209 (19.0)	1098
All ages	680 (16.2)	830 (19.8)	4185	747 (9.9)	1178 (15.7)	7516

reporting long-term extreme fatigue irrespective of previous experience, in the different age and parity groups. Primiparae still reported higher rates within each age band, re-confirming that this was not an 'acceptance' artefact.

Marital status and breast feeding

Unmarried women and breast-feeding women both reported more fatigue. Unmarried women were less likely to breast feed (see Appendix 2, Table A2.3), so that each association might partly mask the other, but discriminant analyses returned both factors as independent predictors. Among married women 12.9% of breast feeders reported fatigue compared with 9.7% of bottle feeders; among unmarried women, 16.8% and 11.6%. There are plausible explanations for both of these associations, similar to those proposed for depression.

Obstetric and anaesthetic predictors

Duration of first stage of labour

The association between long-term extreme fatigue and a long first-stage of labour matched the results for depression. We carried out additional tabulations for different age and parity combinations (Table 13.10) and found that the relationship was not uniform. For multiparae of all ages and for primiparae under age 30 the association was limited to first stage labours of ten hours or more. But for older primiparae, the rates were high for any duration of two hours or more. Although this subgroup-analysis helps to locate the duration-effect, it brings us little closer to a unified explanation. We suggested in relation to depression that since the women themselves designate the onset of the first stage, an early declaration may self-select the same women who are most likely to report symptoms afterwards. This may be part of the explanation here, too.

TABLE 13.10

Extreme tiredness, duration of first stage, parity and age (vaginal deliveries only)

Duration	Primiparae				Multiparae			
	Under 30 yrs		30 yrs or more		Under 30 yrs		30 yrs or more	
	Tired No. (%)	Total women	Tired No. (%)	Total women	Tired No. (%)	Total women	Tired No. (%)	Total women
Under 2 hrs	32 (13.4)	239	10 (14.3)	70	75 (8.4)	890	89 (10.4)	855
2-5 hrs 59 mins	193 (14.3)	1350	92 (23.4)	394	167 (9.2)	1822	172 (10.1)	1698
6-9 hrs 59 mins	101 (14.2)	709	49 (21.3)	230	40 (10.2)	393	39 (11.1)	352
10 hours or more	49 (18.2)	269	18 (20.0)	90	12 (14.0)	86	11 (16.7)	66

Post-partum haemorrhage

The relationship between post-partum haemorrhage (a blood loss in excess of 500 mls) and extreme tiredness was an unexpected finding. There is of course a plausible explanation; it is presumably mediated through subsequent anaemia. The relationship was sub-tabulated (Table 13.11) for the different parity and age groups (shown diagramatically in Figure 13.4) and according to the type of delivery (Figure 13.5). These show that an excess of post-bleed fatigue was present among all the sub-groups, except for the younger primiparae. The highest rates were after vaginal deliveries of first babies in women aged thirty or more. Here, after a post-partum haemorrhage, 36.6% said that they had suffered from extreme fatigue.

Various complications of the puerperium are recorded in the maternity case-notes, one of which is anaemia with a haemoglobin level of less than 10gms per 100mls. There were 504 women (4.3%) with this coding. There was an overlap between a record of anaemia and a post-partum haemorrhage: 224 women had both. But of these two factors it was specifically the post-partum haemorrhage rather than recorded anaemia that was associated with a high risk of fatigue. For the women without a record of anaemia there was no indication as to whether their haemoglobin was higher than 10 gms, or whether in fact it was not measured.

Figure 13.4 Fatigue, PPH, Parity and Age

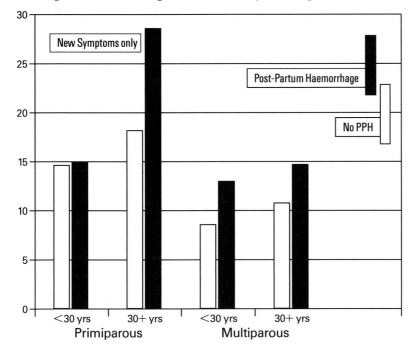

TABLE 13.11

Extreme tiredness, post-partum haemorrhage parity, age and type of delivery

	Primiparae				Multiparae			
	Under 30 yrs		30 yrs or more		Under 30 yrs		30 yrs or more	
	Tired	Total	Tired	Total	Tired	Total	Tired	Total
	No. (%)	women	No. (%)	women	No. (%)	women	No. (%)	women
Vaginal deliveries								
Post-partum haemorrhage	39 (13.9)	281	37 (36.6)	101	22 (13.0)	169	22 (15.6)	141
No post-partum haemorrhage	339 (14.6)	2322	135 (19.5)	691	276 (8.8)	3134	297 (10.1)	2947
Caesarean sections								
Post-partum haemorrhage	35 (16.4)	213	26 (21.3)	122	25 (12.9)	194	38 (14.2)	266
No post-partum haemorrhage	41 (15.2)	269	28 (15.1)	186	19 (7.1)	268	48 (12.1)	397

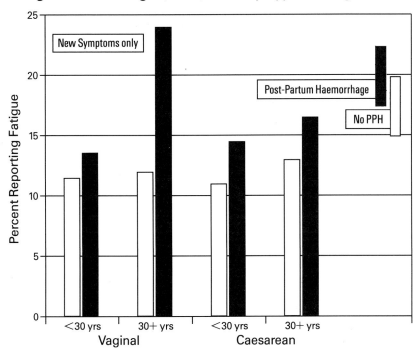

Figure 13.5   Fatigue, PPH, Delivery-Type and Age

Inhalation analgesia

The predictive effect of inhalation analgesia (pre-mixed 50/50 nitrous oxide and oxygen) used for pain relief, upon the rates of fatigue, was another unexpected finding. This is more difficult to explain. This form of pain relief is generally regarded as harmless. Discriminant analysis should have compensated for any direct associations through parity or age, but we sub-tabulated the relationship among the different parity and age groups (Table 13.12). Figure 13.6 demonstrates this diagramtically. The increased rates of extreme tiredness after inhalation analgesia were evident in both parity groups but, like post-partum haemorrhage, more striking among women aged thirty or more. This brings us no closer to a suggested mechanism.

We considered the possibility of a drug specific self-selection process such that women with a predisposition towards tiredness demand inhalation analgesia more readily; but it seemed implausible, and we could find no corroborative evidence within the data set or in the literature. We then questioned whether nitrous oxide might be toxic, and found some evidence on this point. Studies, in animals under prolonged exposure, have established a pharmacological interference mechanism between nitrous oxide and vitamin B_{12} metabolism.

TABLE 13.12

Extreme tiredness, inhalation analgesia*, parity and age

	Primiparae				Multiparae			
	Under 30 yrs		30 yrs or more		Under 30 yrs		30 yrs or more	
	Tired	Total	Tired	Total	Tired	Total	Tired	Total
	No. (%)	women	No. (%)	women	No. (%)	women	No. (%)	women
Inhalation	204 (15.5)	1318	87 (24.5)	355	175 (10.0)	1749	181 (12.1)	1494
No inhalation	250 (14.1)	1767	139 (18.7)	745	167 (8.3)	2016	224 (9.9)	2257

*Pre-mixed 50/50 nitrous oxide and oxygen

Figure 13.6 Fatigue, Inhalation*, Parity and Age

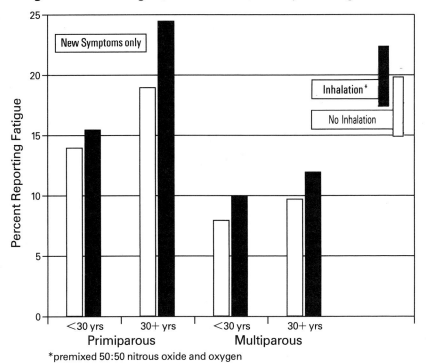

*premixed 50:50 nitrous oxide and oxygen

What predicts onsets and durations of extreme tiredness?

Although our main analyses were confined to first-time extreme tiredness, starting within the first three months, and lasting any time over six weeks, we also analysed different onsets and durations within and outside these limits.

Different predictive factors were related to different onset-times (Table 13.13). Maternal age, breast feeding, multiple pregnancy and post-partum haemorrhage predicted tiredness starting within the first week, but not of later onset. Primiparity and a long first-stage were related more widely to onsets within the first four weeks. However, non-married women showed no excess of early onsets, but only of fatigue beginning two to thirteen weeks after delivery. Inhalation analgesia was different again, predicting tiredness starting two to four weeks after delivery. Subsidiary discriminant analyses of different onsets confirmed these observations.

193

TABLE 13.13

Differing onsets of extreme tiredness and main predictors

	Onset Within 1 week No. %	2 – 4 weeks No. %	5 – 13 weeks No. %	3 – 12 months No. %	Total women
Parity					
Primiparae	521 (12.45)	100 (2.39)	59 (1.41)	52 (1.24)	4185
Multiparae	518 (6.89)	130 (1.73)	99 (1.32)	116 (1.54)	7516
Relative risks	1.81	1.38	1.07(NS)	0.81(NS)	
Age					
Under 30 years	571 (8.34)	138 (2.01)	87 (1.27)	108 (1.58)	6850
30 years or more	468 (9.65)	92 (1.90)	71 (1.46)	70 (1.44)	4851
Relative risks	1.16	0.95(NS)	1.15(NS)	0.91(NS)	
Marital status					
Married	920 (8.74)	200 (1.90)	135 (1.28)	156 (1.48)	10525
Single	119 (10.12)	30 (2.55)	23 (1.96)	22 (1.87)	1176
Relative risks	1.16(NS)	1.34	1.53	1.26(NS)	
Type of feeding					
Breast	782 (9.85)	163 (2.05)	107 (1.35)	121 (1.52)	7937
Artificial	257 (6.83)	67 (1.78)	51 (1.35)	58 (1.54)	3764
Relative risks	1.44	1.15(NS)	1.0(NS)	0.99(NS)	
Multiple pregnancy					
Multiple	26 (15.38)	8 (4.73)		2 (1.18)	169
Singleton	1031 (8.78)	380 (3.30)		177 (1.53)	11532
Relative risks	1.75	1.43(NS)		0.77(NS)	
1st stage labour					
Under 6 hours	588 (8.03)	142 (1.94)	100 (1.37)	105 (1.43)	7318
6 hours or more	239 (10.89)	51 (2.32)	29 (1.32)	40 (1.82)	2195
Relative risks	1.36	1.20(NS)	1.04(NS)	1.27(NS)	
Post-partum haemorrhage					
PPH	181 (12.17)	27 (1.82)	8 (0.54)	18 (1.21)	1487
No PPH	858 (8.4)	194 (1.90)	131 (1.28)	160 (1.57)	10214
Relative risks	1.45	0.96(NS)	0.42(NS)	0.77(NS)	
Inhalation					
Inhalation	462 (9.40)	112 (2.28)	73 (1.48)	70 (1.42)	4916
No inhalation	577 (8.50)	118 (1.74)	85 (1.25)	108 (1.59)	6785
Relative risk	1.11(NS)	1.31	1.18(NS)	0.89(NS)	

Reports of fatigue with different durations are examined in Table 13.14. Unlike similar analyses of many other health problems the different durations exhibited several distinctive associations. The most striking was for post-partum haemorrhage, with a much greater relative risk among symptoms of short duration and with no increased risk for symptoms lasting more than twelve months. Inhalation analgesia was associated only with symptoms of intermediate duration of three to twelve months. These two factors, and their comparable onset-associations are compatible with the separate anaemia-generating mechanisms postulated. All these relationships were confirmed through discriminant analysis.

Unmarried status and greater maternal age predicted extreme tiredness only of the longest duration, symptoms still persisting at the time of the enquiry. Multiple pregnancy predicted tiredness lasting over a year. These world observations would accord with the presumed mechanisms – social, domestic and economic pressures, lack of sleep and extra physical work.

Combined symptoms

Depression and tiredness were strongly inter-related. Almost half the women with first-time depression (496) reported first-time extreme tiredness as well. We compared the separate associations of the combined symptoms with each of the two alone. Detailed tabulations for each, with calculated crude relative risks are given in Tables 13.15 and 13.16 and later we undertook separate discriminant analyses.

These analyses provided several additional findings of note. The first was an association between depression alone and earlier maternal age, which had not been evident in the analysis of depression with or without fatique (Table 13.15). The age association for fatigue was in the opposite direction to that for depression. Primiparae had more of each symptom but the association for depression alone was marginal and not independently significant on discriminant analysis. These parity and age relationships remained after allowing for the possible artefactual effect of our acceptance-restriction to first-time symptoms.

A negative association with Asian ethnic group became evident for depression alone; while the relationship with breast feeding was present in the 'fatigue' groups, but not for depression alone (Table 13.16). The associations with post-partum haemorrhage and inhalation were confirmed as being related to straightforward tiredness only. Twins were associated with higher symptom rates in all three groups. Finally, both unmarried status and smaller babies were independent predictors of the combined symptoms only. These additional points had not been visible without this combined form of analysis.

TABLE 13.14

Differing durations of extreme tiredness and main predictors

	Duration 6 weeks-3 months No. (%)	3 – 6 months No. (%)	6 – 12 months No. (%)	Over 12 months No. (%)	Still persistent No. (%)	Total women
Parity						
Primiparae	109 (2.6)	141 (3.37)	126 (3.01)	61 (1.46)	243 (5.81)	4185
Multiparae	72 (0.96)	130 (1.73)	124 (1.65)	110 (1.46)	311 (4.14)	7516
Relative risks	2.71	1.95	1.82	1.0 (NS)	1.40	
Age						
Under 30 years	101 (1.47)	163 (2.38)	147 (2.15)	92 (1.34)	293 (4.28)	6850
30 years or more	80 (1.65)	108 (2.22)	103 (2.12)	79 (1.63)	261 (5.38)	4851
Relative risks	1.12(NS)	0.93(NS)	0.99(NS)	1.22(NS)	1.26	
Marital status						
Married	165 (1.57)	242 (2.3)	228 (2.17)	161 (1.53)	459 (4.36)	10525
Non-married	16 (1.36)	29 (2.47)	22 (1.87)	10 (0.85)	95 (8.08)	1176
Relative risks	0.87(NS)	1.07(NS)	0.86(NS)	0.56(NS)	1.85	
Type of feeding						
Breast	142 (1.79)	201 (2.53)	194 (2.44)	124 (1.56)	391 (4.93)	7937
Artificial	39 (1.04)	70 (1.86)	56 (1.49)	47 (1.25)	163 (4.33)	3764
Relative risks	1.72	1.36	1.64	1.25(NS)	1.01(NS)	
Multiple pregnancy						
Multiple	2 (1.18)	6 (3.55)	5 (2.96)	6 (3.55)	15 (8.88)	169
Singleton	179 (1.55)	265 (2.30)	245 (2.12)	165 (1.43)	539 (4.67)	11532
Relative risks	1.55	1.29(NS)	2.12	2.48	1.90	

TABLE 13.14 Cont.

	Duration 6 weeks- 3 months No. (%)	3 – 6 months No. (%)	6 – 12 months No. (%)	Over 12 months No. (%)	Still persistent No. (%)	Total women
1st stage labour						
Under 6 hours	99 (1.35)	161 (2.20)	142 (1.94)	105 (1.43)	323 (4.41)	7318
6 hours or more	43 (1.96)	60 (2.73)	48 (2.19)	43 (1.96)	125 (5.69)	2195
Relative risks	1.45	1.24(NS)	1.13(NS)	1.37(NS)	1.29	
Post-partum haemorrhage						
PPH	48 (3.23)	44 (2.96)	40 (2.69)	24 (1.61)	88 (5.92)	1487
No PPH	133 (1.30)	227 (2.22)	210 (2.06)	147 (1.44)	466 (4.56)	10214
Relative risks	2.56	1.33	1.31	1.12(NS)	1.30*	
Inhalation						
Inhalation	77 (1.57)	128 (2.60)	119 (2.42)	79 (1.60)	244 (4.96)	4916
No inhalation	104 (1.53)	143 (2.11)	131 (1.93)	92 (1.38)	310 (4.57)	6785
Relative risks	1.03(NS)	1.23	1.25	1.18(NS)	1.09(NS)	

*Not statistically significant on discriminant analysis

TABLE 13.15

Combination of depression and extreme tiredness, age and parity

Maternal Age	Primiparae				Multiparae			
	Just depression No. (%)	Just tiredness No. (%)	Both symptoms No. (%)	Total women	Just depression No. (%)	Just tiredness No. (%)	Both symptoms No. (%)	Total women
Under 25 years	113 (7.3)	116 (7.4)	81 (5.2)	1558	61 (5.7)	56 (5.2)	36 (3.4)	1067
25 – 29 years	78 (5.1)	165 (10.8)	92 (6.0)	1527	115 (4.3)	156 (5.8)	94 (3.5)	2698
30 – 34 years	51 (6.3)	106 (13.1)	58 (7.2)	810	105 (4.0)	189 (7.1)	76 (2.9)	2653
35 years or more	11 (3.8)	39 (13.4)	23 (7.9)	290	35 (3.2)	104 (9.5)	36 (3.3)	1098
All ages	253 (6.1)	426 (10.2)	254 (6.1)	4185	316 (4.2)	505 (6.7)	242 (3.2)	7516

TABLE 13.16

Combined symptoms and main predictors

	Just depression	Just tiredness	Both	Total women
	No. (%)	No. (%)	No. (%)	
Married	492 (4.67)	830 (7.89)	425 (4.04)	10525
Unmarried	77 (6.55)	101 (8.59)	71 (6.04)	1176
Relative risks	1.40*	1.09(NS)	1.50	
Caucasian	501 (4.94)	825 (8.14)	435 (4.29)	10135
Asian	15 (2.83)	28 (5.28)	23 (4.34)	530
Relative risks	1.75	1.54*	0.99	
Twins	11 (6.51)	23 (13.61)	11 (6.51)	169
Singleton	558 (4.84)	908 (7.87)	485 (4.21)	11532
Relative risks	1.35**	1.73	1.55*	
Breast feeding	385 (4.85)	688 (8.67)	364 (4.59)	7937
Artificial feeding	184 (4.89)	243 (6.46)	132 (3.51)	3764
Relative risks	0.99(NS)	1.34	1.31	
PPH	85 (5.72)	165 (11.10)	79 (5.31)	1487
No PPH	484 (4.74)	766 (7.50)	417 (4.08)	10214
Relative risks	1.21(NS)	1.48	1.30*	
Inhalation	214 (4.35)	435 (8.85)	212 (4.31)	4916
No inhalation	355 (5.23)	496 (7.31)	284 (4.19)	6785
Relative risks	0.83(NS)	1.21	1.03(NS)	
Weight up to 3200 grams	230 (5.25)	338 (7.72)	213 (4.86)	4380
3201 grams or more	339 (4.63)	593 (8.10)	283 (3.87)	7321
Relative risk	1.13(NS)	0.95(NS)	1.26	

*These, although significantly different here, were **not** independent predictors after discriminant analysis.

These, although not statistically significant here, **were independent predictors after discriminant analysis.

Discussion

Depression and tiredness are well recognised problems after childbirth. They can be related: fatique and sleeplessness may contribute to depression while depression can lead to sleeplessness and fatigue. Depression has been much studied, with more published work than for any of the other health problems investigated in this study. However, we found no published investigations of extreme fatigue per se.

Prevalence estimates of post-partum depression in different investigations have ranged from 3% up to 30%, depending upon the definitions and durations used, and the timings, of the assessments (Tod 1964; Gordon et al 1965; Gelder 1978; Kumar and Robson 1984). A recent estimate in this country suggests around 10%, as a working estimate (Brockington and Cox-Roper 1988). Our own minimum estimate was that 9.1% of the women suffered new long-term depression, although the inclusion of continuing or recurrent symptoms raises this to 13.4%. These estimates are based upon all well-dated cases of depression/anxiety occurring within three months of the delivery and persisting for more than six weeks. Few published estimates have distinguished between new and recurrent symptoms.

Previous studies have shown that although post-partum depression can continue for long periods, the majority of cases subside within a year (Brandon 1983; Gelder 1978). This was confirmed here; 60% of the 1065 new occurrences of depression had resolved within this period. Nevertheless, 27% of cases (284) were reported to be still unresolved by the time of our enquiry, thirteen months to nine years after the birth.

Tiredness after giving birth and looking after a baby is to be expected and is probably universal. However its prevalence in an extreme form over longer periods is not documented. In this population 17.1% reported extreme tiredness, as they perceived it, occurring within three months of delivery and persisting for more than six weeks: among them, 12.2% had never before had tiredness so extreme; and for 6.1% it persisted for more than a year.

Our questionnaire was not designed to distinguish clearly between post-partum depression and anxiety states. Reporting depended upon self-perception, and upon the manner of labelling by the woman or by a doctor – although the first is anyway a critical determinant of the last. Nevertheless, the approach offered two important advantages. First, it gathered data from an unusually large number of women; most other studies of postnatal depression have been based upon smaller samples. Second, it accessed a great deal of linkable delivery-related data. These two features together allowed us to avoid some of the ambiguities which have arisen in other studies, from numerical inadequacy and internal complexities, and which in turn have led to so wide a variety of reported conclusions.

For example, some investigators have found post-partum depression to be more common after a first birth (Wilson et al 1972; Bridge et al 1985); some after a subsequent birth (Tod 1964); while others have found no parity relationship (Cox et al 1982). Some linked depression with early maternal age (Paykel et al 1980; Feggetter and Gath 1981) while others have found no age relationship (Jacobson et al 1965). We ourselves found a marginal but non-independent excess of depression among first births, and we found more depression, occurring without fatigue, among younger mothers (under 25 years). Older mothers, at all parities, had more extreme fatigue; but older primiparae had higher rates than any other group.

Some investigators have found unmarried status to be linked to postnatal depression (Feggetter and Garth 1981), but others have found no association (Cox et al, 1982, Watson et al 1984). In our own investigation this was an important predictor of depression accompanied by fatigue, and of chronic unresolved symptoms. If we could have separated non-married women living with a partner, and those who had married by the time of the birth, from those who lived alone, the rates of depression and tiredness among the last group might have been greater still.

Breast feeding at the time of discharge from hospital was associated with fatigue with or without depression, but not of depression alone. It predicted only the immediate onset shorter duration symptoms. Case-note data on breast feeding at discharge is an unsatisfactory indicator: many women give up breast feeding soon afterwards and an investigation of women who continued to breast feed is needed. Continuing breast feeders might be less depressed because of their success in feeding: or more depressed because of the additional burdens, ties and sleeplessness that breast feeding entails. Other investigations have found a relationship between infant feeding and postnatal depression. Dalton (1971), in a study of fourteen depressed mothers (all requiring treatment), and 175 non-depressed mothers, found that breast feeding at two weeks was associated with depression. Adler and Cox (1983) compared full and partial breast feeding with bottle feeding, at twelve weeks, and found more depression among those fully breast feeding. In both investigations however the numbers were small.

Obstetric and delivery procedures have been examined in other studies of postnatal depression and some have shown positive relationships (Oakley 1980; Kumar and Robson 1984; Jacoby 1987); while others have not (Pitt 1968; Martin 1977; Playfair and Gowers 1981; Kendall et al, 1981; O'Hara et al 1982). Particular procedures implicated here have included inductions, Caesarean section, forceps delivery and epidural anaesthesia. Some special interest groups (such as the National Childbirth Trust) have related depression to deprivation of personal autonomy, with obstetric interventions resulting in a 'loss of control' of the birth process.

We ourselves found that only a Caesarean section among the obstetric procedures was followed by an increased rate of depression; and this was despite the proven predictive power of the other procedures in relation to other symptoms. Even with Caesarean section, the association with depression was not uniform; it was present only among women giving birth to their first child. The other obstetric associations of depression related to the circumstances and processes of childbirth, rather than the procedures, a long first-stage of labour, twins and lower birthweight.

Twins were associated with depression and with fatigue, especially those complaints lasting more than twelve months. The association with twins does not seem to have been recorded in the literature, possibly because most studies had insufficient numbers. It is an understandable connection, probably operating through the extra burdens of caring for twins, including lack of sleep. The delivery of a smaller baby was also related to depression and fatigue, and especially together. Additional 'burden-of-care' effects could again provide an explanation.

There were two more delivery factors which predicted extreme tiredness occurring without depression: post-partum haemorrhage, and inhalation nitrous-oxide analgesia. The fatigue associated with a post-partum haemorrhage began in the first post-delivery week and was relatively short-lived, a sequence compatible with a sudden lowering of haemoglobin levels and a gradual replenishment: we postulate that this fatigue results from anaemia. The early discharge of women after delivery might mean that many women do not have their haemoglobin measured at all; while others might be measured before post haemorrhage haemodilution has taken place. Those who are found to have anaemia are given a short supply of treatment and the general practitioner is expected to replenish this where necessary; this may not always occur. In addition to a possible failure in the detection of anaemia, this is another point at which the system can break down. Women rarely have any contact with the maternity services after their six-week postnatal examination and even then haemoglobin measurement is not always carried out. Many women would expect their tiredness to have 'non-medical' causes and would not initiate a special visit to the doctor. Whatever the reason it seems likely that a number of women have undiagnosed and/or untreated post-partum anaemia. If confirmed, this particular problem is easily remediable, and further investigation and action are clearly necessary.

The association between inhalation analgesia and fatigue, closely resembling that following post-partum haemorrhage, led us to search the literature for anaemia-producing effects of nitrous oxide. We found evidence that nitrous oxide can interfere with vitamin B_{12} metabolism (Baden et al 1984; Koblin and Tomerson 1990). The expected form of subsequent anaemia is exactly compatible with the timing of the fatique symptoms, namely an intermediate onset and recovery not long drawn-out. However, these toxicological studies were based mainly on animals and we must be extremely cautious about our interpretations. As with post-partum haemorrhage, further investigation is needed, especially since if there were a vitamin B_{12} link there is a ready solution to the problem.

The reporting of depression and extreme tiredness, more than most symptoms included in this investigation, are likely to relate to variations in individual perceptions. What some women will report as fatigue others will report as depression and others will not report at all. Medical consultation rates for depression were greater than for fatigue, and this may in part reflect the effects of medical labelling; although attendance may in the first place reflect the mother's initial perception. Perceptual variations may also explain the high rates of reported extreme tiredness among older primiparae compared with multiparae of the same age. Women who have already had one child will expect fatigue, regard it as normal, and not report it; but a new mother especially an older one, might find the whole experience more of a shock. The associations between unmarried status, and depression combined with fatigue, could also reflect perceptual variations influenced by the social context.

Nonetheless many of the findings of this investigation are readily interpretable. In particular they can be related to indicators of inadequate levels of social support and a more stressful post-partum environment. There are obvious additional 'burdens-of-care' likely in women who are unmarried and who live alone, who have twins or a small baby, and who breast feed, especially for long periods. The lower rate of depression in Asian women is also compatible with the community support and extended family groups more typical in this ethnic sub-culture. The findings of this study do not generally provide evidence to suggest that obstetric or anaesthetic interventions have a major determining role in relation to postnatal depression.

Chapter 14 – Less Frequent Symptoms

We enquired about several symptoms and diagnoses not so far discussed in detail. They included bowel upsets, indigestion, dental problems, buzzing in ears, visual disturbances, dizziness or fainting, high blood pressure and varicose veins. In addition to these specified symptoms there was an 'open' question, asking the women to note any others not in the primary list. All of the specified symptoms were relatively infrequent, reported only by small numbers of women, and ranging from 2.7% for bowel upsets, to 0.4% for high blood pressure. The frequencies are shown in Table 14.1. The first column gives the numbers and proportions of women experiencing newly-occurring symptoms, starting within three months of delivery and lasting for more than six weeks. The second column includes recurrent but otherwise similar symptoms – those which had also been experienced before.

Some of these questions – hypertension, varicose veins – were included because of their intrinsic interest: but others had been included chiefly for 'control' purposes, and as 'negative checks'.

The first 'control' purpose related to the original objective of the study, our investigations of the possible long-term effects of epidural anaesthesia. Neither

TABLE 14.1

Frequencies of symptoms

Symptom	No. (%) newly occurring within 3 mths – over 6 wks	No. (%) including recurrences
Bowel upsets	321 (2.7)	550 (5.7)
Indigestion	127 (1.1)	409 (3.5)
Dental problems	124 (1.1)	316 (2.7)
Buzzing in ears	76 (0.6)	170 (1.5)
Flashing lights/ spots before eyes	174 (1.5)	467 (4.0)
Dizziness/fainting	211 (1.8)	406 (3.5)
High blood pressure	48 (0.4)	208 (1.8)
Varicose veins	151 (1.3)	862 (7.4)
Other (specified by woman)	423 (3.6)	555 (4.7)

the questionnaire, nor the accompanying letter gave any hint that epidurals, or indeed any other type of pain relief or obstetric procedure, were the subject of particular enquiry. However, we had to test the possibility that an anticipation of side-effects by the women or that subsequent anxieties could lead to a general over-reporting of all symptoms.

Our second 'control' necessity was an extension of the first. We needed an indicator of 'neuroticism'. This was partly to 'tag' and thus exclude particular respondents whose indiscriminate over-reporting might invalidate our analyses and conclusions: and partly to provide a basis for assessing the validity of other questions and the reponses to them. We also needed to 'control' the possibility that women with a tendency to over-report might also preferentially 'acquire' certain obstetric procedures, or be more liable to particular obstetric complications – epidurals or long labours, for example – and thus to 'create' spurious connections with subsequently reported symptoms. The questions directed particularly towards this end related to buzzing in the ears, visual disturbances and dizziness or fainting; although other symptoms discussed in previous chapters – tingling in hands and feet, headache, depression/anxiety and extreme fatigue – might also sometimes be relevant in this connection.

The 'open' question also served two main purposes. First, it allowed a measure of the frequencies of uncommon health problems and an assessment of their relationships with obstetric or social factors; and second, it might supply additional 'control' material.

Hypertension

Hypertension during pregnancy is relatively common. It can occur as essential or chronic hypertension but it is more frequently specific to pregnancy when it is referred to as gestational or pregnancy-induced hypertension. It is also a consequence of the pregnancy-specific-disease, pre-eclampsia, in which hypertension is combined with proteinuria. It has been suggested that gestational hypertension is an early indicator, in some women, of later essential hypertension; or that pregnancy can act as an immediate trigger for the development of essential hypertension, which then continues into the post-partum period (Llewellyn-Jones 1990). Classically, gestational hypertension recovers immediately after delivery and this has often been regarded as part of its definition, but in some women blood pressure continues to be raised for a time after delivery, before eventually subsiding. There is however no quantitative documentation in the literature of the proportions of women in whom this occurs, nor of its duration when it does.

In the maternity case-notes the general category of 'hypertension' included separate codes for essential hypertension; gestational hypertension; proteinuria more than trace; severe pre-eclampsia; and eclampsia. A total of 1055 women had one or more of these codes. There were 86 coded as having essential or chronic hypertension, 19 of whom had gestational hypertension superimposed. Since we would expect essential hypertension to continue after delivery, these 86 were excluded from the follow-up analyses. Of the remaining 969 women (6% of the sample), 714 were coded as having gestational hypertension without note of other signs of pre-eclampsia; 140 had gestational hypertension with proteinuria; and 42 women were recorded as having severe pre-eclampsia, with admission to intensive care. The last 182, with varying severities of pre-eclampsia, represented 1.6% of the sample. The remaining 73 women were coded as having proteinuria but with no hypertension. We could not tell if they were mis-coded with unrecorded gestational hypertension, so we have kept them as a separate follow-up group.

There were 208 (1.8%) questionnaire reports of high blood pressure occurring after the delivery and lasting for more than six weeks. This included 51 of the 714 women (7.1%) with straightforward gestational hypertension; 22 of the 182 women (12.%) with proteinuric hypertension and 7 of the 73 women (9.6%) coded as having proteinuria without hypertension. In over 50% (41) of these 80 reported instances of continued hypertension (similar proportions in each category) high blood pressure was still present at the time of our enquiry, thirteen months to nine years later. The remaining (128) reports of post-delivery hypertension were in women who had no record of hypertension during the index pregnancy.

There was information from the questionnaires about treatment and referral. Among the 22 women with raised blood pressure continuing after proteinuric hypertension, 15 (68%) said they were given tablets for this by their general practitioner, which tends to confirm that the doctors also thought that the high blood pressure had continued; but none were referred for specialist consultation. This lack of referral in this group might explain why a continuation of hypertension following pre-eclampsia has not been generally recognised. Our conclusion is that the matter should be investigated, and the problem reviewed on the basis of more carefully ascertained antenatal and post-partum diagnoses.

Varicose veins

Many women experience varicose veins in association with pregnancy and childbirth. They generally appear during the course of the pregnancy rather than following the delivery of the child. They are believed to become worse with each successive pregnancy and can become permanent. (Hibbard 1988; Llewellyn-Jones 1990).

Only 151 women (1.3%) reported varicose veins complying with our general 'acceptance-criteria' as new symptoms starting within three months of the index delivery, and persisting for longer than six weeks. A much larger number (711, 6.1%) reported varicose veins of similar duration which had first occurred at some time before the delivery. Some no doubt occurred during a previous pregnancy, some during the index pregnancy and some would be unrelated to pregnancy. Some would have worsened by stages. We cannot systematically distinguish between these classes, but 69 of the 711 women (9.7%) said spontaneously that their varicose veins had first occurred during an earlier pregnancy and 111 (15.6%) said they had started during the index pregnancy. Seventy-three women said that although they had had varicose veins before, they were much worse since the birth.

Discriminant analysis of the 151 new cases of long-term post-partum varicose veins was carried out in order to identify any independent obstetric or social predictors. None at all were found.

We repeated the discrimination exercise including recurrences and continuations of varicose veins as well as new occurrences. Three maternal factors then appeared as independent predictors: multiparity, increased maternal age, and greater maternal height. The proportions of symptoms by parity ranged from 5.2% of para-0 women; 8.3% of para-1 women; 9.8% of para-2; 11.6% of para-3; 12.3% of para-4 to 16.8% of para-5+. Proportions by age ranged from 3.6% at age under 20; 4.8% of ages 20-24; 6.7% of ages 25-29; 9.2% of ages 30-34; to 10.2% of ages 35+. These findings suggest a pregnancy acquisition or worsening under both criteria. Maternal height also exhibited an independent linear association. Among women under 150 cms in height, 3.8% reported varicose veins, compared with 5.4% of those between 150 and 159 cms; 8.1% between 160 and 169 cms; and 10.3% for 170 cms or taller. This association is not easily interpreted – unless it represents the effects of hydrostatic pressure – but it parallels the (crude) association already reported between height and haemorrhoids.

This symptom sheds some light on our concern about the possible inclusion on the part of the women of symptoms starting in pregnancy. Among the whole group of women with long-term post-partum varicose veins, a particularly high proportion (83%) had said that they were not new symptoms. Since this complaint is typically initiated in pregnancy, this is what we would expect: it suggests that most women had understood our questionnaire instructions accurately and had interpreted pregnancy-induced varicose veins as having occurred *before* the birth.

Bowel upsets, indigestion and dental problems

We included in the questionnaire some deliberately vague questions on 'bowel upsets', 'indigestion' and 'dental problems'. this was chiefly to assist in our assessment of the effects of epidural anaesthesia. If an association had been found between these three symptoms and this procedure, we would have had to reconsider the validity of any other recorded associations. In fact there were no associations between epidural anaesthesia and any of these complaints.

Discriminant analysis, seeking other independent symptom predictors, showed that for indigestion and for dental problems a longer first stage of labour was the only one. We noted earlier that the onset of the first stage of labour is generally designated by the women, and some will define the onset with relatively mild contractions. A longer 'duration' might also reflect a tendency to report more trivial conditions: these relationships possibly exhibit the common consequences of a particular personality type.

'Bowel upsets' were predicted by early maternal age, forceps delivery and a longer second stage labour. The age relationship seemed to be a selective artefact arising from our 'inclusion criteria', but the other two predictors were the same as we had found for haemorrhoids. There were 67 women who reported haemorrhoids as well as bowel upsets: this amounted to 21% of the bowel upset group. Some women were clearly labelling haemorrhoids additionally under this second heading, and many gave the same times of onset, durations, previous histories, medical consultations and treatments for both reported symptoms. Other women might have mis-labelled haemorrhoids as bowel upsets and reported them instead under this alternative category.

We conducted a special discriminant analysis for bowel upsets including haemorrhoids as a confounding factor, in order to see if the associations with forceps and long second stage would disappear. The long labour effect did, which would confirm an explanation in terms of double-labelling. However the forceps association remained highly significant. We have since speculated whether faecal incontinence – not on our list of symptoms – associated with perineal trauma, might have been entered under this heading. This is a question which needs to be pursued on another occasion.

'Indigestion' may also have attracted unintended entries. We had noted earlier (Table 7.3) that many reports of indigestion were timed to the first post-partum week, and we wondered if some women may have been referring to the 'heartburn' of later pregnancy rather than indigestion first starting after the delivery.

Buzzing in ears, visual disturbance, dizziness or fainting

These particular symptoms were also included initially for 'control' purposes, as indicators of 'hypochondria' or 'neuroticism'. As expected, reports of the three symptoms were inter-correlated. However, and to our surprise, they also showed strong relationships with several of the social, obstetric and anaesthetic factors. Some, but not all, turned out to represent cross-associations between these reported symptoms and migraine.

Buzzing in the ears, within our standard symptom acceptance criteria, was reported by only 76 (0.6%) women. It was a long-lasting problem, with 55 of these women (72%) still complaining of it at the time of the enquiry. Less than half of the 76 (41%) had consulted a doctor; 13 received treatment, and a further 7 were referred. Discriminant analyses revealed three positive independent predictors of buzzing in the ears: Asian ethnic group ($F = 15.370$); lower

TABLE 14.2

Visual disturbances, migraine and relationships with symptom predictors

	Just visual disturbances	Just migraine	Both symptoms	Total women
	No. (%)	No. (%)	No. (%)	
Epidural	62 (1.30)	71 (1.49)	21 (0.44)	4766
No epidural	79 (1.14)	61 (0.88)	12 (0.17)	6935
Pethidine	29 (1.75)	21 (1.27)	4 (0.24)	1658
No pethidine	112 (1.12)	111 (1.11)	29 (0.29)	10043
General anaesthesia	20 (1.73)	12 (1.04)	6 (0.52)	1158
No general anaesthesia	121 (1.15)	120 (1.14)	27 (0.26)	10543
Spinal	5 (3.13)	2 (1.25)	1 (0.63)	160
No spinal	136 (1.18)	130 (1.13)	32 (0.28)	11541

birthweight (F = 4.2731); general anaesthesia (but not Caesarean section independently) (F = 5.4270). Since these findings are all based on small numbers they require confirmation.

Visual disturbances, described on the questionnaire as 'flashing lights or spots before the eyes', were reported by 174 women (1.5%). Like buzzing in the ears they were long lasting, with 67% still persisting. Only 60 of the women (34%) went to the doctor; but 37 of them were given treatment and a further 10 were referred. Discriminant analyses identified several independent predictors of visual disturbances: the use of pethidine (F = 10.825); spinal block (F = 9.1520); epidural anaesthesia (F = 5.1292); and general anaesthesia (F = 8.2692). The use of tranquillisers during early labour was a negative predictor (F = 4.3975). A relationship with early maternal age (F = 6.0334) turned out to be an artefact of our symptom inclusion criteria.

Visual disturbances sometimes occur with migraine, and 33 of the 174 women reported both (Odds Ratio = 20.2). The overlap between these two symptoms led us to re-examine visual disturbances in women who did and did not report migraine (Table 14.2), showing that the epidural relationship was specific to

TABLE 14.3

Dizziness/fainting, migraine and relationship with symptom predictors

	Just dizziness/ fainting	Just migraine	Both symptoms	Total women
	No. (%)	No. (%)	No. (%)	
Epidural	86 (1.80)	76 (1.59)	21 (0.44)	4766
No epidural	98 (1.41)	62 (0.89)	12 (0.17)	6935
General anaesthesia	28 (2.42)	13 (1.12)	5 (0.43)	1158
No general anaesthesia	156 (1.48)	125 (1.19)	22 (0.21)	10543
Spinal	6 (3.75)	3 (1.9)	–	160
No spinal	178 (1.54)	135 (1.17)	27	11541

those visual disturbances which occurred with migraine. A special discriminant analysis of visual disturbances, holding migraine as a confounder, confirmed that the crude relationship between epidural anaesthesia and the risk of visual disturbances then disappeared. However, similar analyses showed that the associations with pethidine, and with general and spinal anaesthesia, remained as specific predictors and were not a result of the migraine interaction.

Dizziness and/or fainting, within the standard symptom inclusion criteria, were reported by 211 women (1.8%). The durations were less than for the previous two symptoms, with only 55% of symptoms still persisting. However greater proportions (50%) consulted a doctor: of these, half were treated and 14% referred for specialist consultation. There were four independent predictors of dizziness/fainting; early maternal age (F = 15.157); epidural anaesthesia (F = 8.5327); general anaesthesia (F = 10.864); and spinal anaesthesia (F = 4.2682).

This symptom was again related to migraine, with 27 women mentioning both symptoms. (Odds Ratio = 12.1). Detailed cross-tabulations, in the same form as for visual disturbances, at first seemed to indicate that the epidural association was restricted to dizziness occurring with migraine (Table 14.3). However a subsidiary discriminant analysis of dizziness/fainting, with migraine entered as a confounder, failed this time to disperse the epidural association. The associations with general and spinal anaesthesia were retained in both analyses. Even the maternal-age association appeared, from a discriminant analysis of new and recurrent symptoms, to be genuine, and not a selection artefact.

Since general anaesthesia was found to be an independent predictor of each of the three symptoms in this group, we tabulated its effect against all of them jointly. Of the 383 women who reported one or more of buzzing in the ears, visual disturbances and dizziness/fainting, 57 had had general anesthesia, giving a significant overall relative risk of 1.36.

Open-question responses

We included at the end of the questionnaire an open question, where the women were asked to note any other health problems which they had experienced. We extracted from these reports, as was now customary, all those problems which had first occurred within three months of the index delivery and had persisted for more than six weeks. A total of 423 women (3.6%) reported at least one symptom and some specified more than one, to give 449 all together. The individual symptoms were all infrequently reported but might have included relatively more serious conditions, since there was a high rate of GP consultation (68%).

In order to permit formal analysis of this open category we devised a form of categorisation which accounted for 70% of all of the symptoms, as follows;

Menstrual problems	57
Perineal problems	53
Numbness/tingling/loss of sensation	37
Mood disturbances	36
Thrush and other genital infections	32
Prolapse and related symptoms	26
Arthritis/joint pains	19
Abdominal pain	17
Skin problems	14
Hair loss	7
Weight problems	7
Urinary tract infections	7
All others	137

Menstrual problems of various types were the most frequently reported symptoms in the open question, and included heavy and/or irregular periods, in 40 women: and pre-menstrual tension (PMT) in 17 women. These problems were generally persistent, with 68% still present at the time of our enquiry. Most affected women (65%) had consulted their doctors, and of the 37 who consulted, 10 (27%) were referred for specialist consultation. Pre-menstrual tension was however exceptional in this respect; of 14 consulting a doctor, none were referred. The non-PMT menstrual problems (85%) were mostly in multiparae but PMT was evenly distributed between primiparae and multiparae.

Perineal problems of various kinds were reported by 53 women and included complaints described as; 'painful perineum'; 'pain during intercourse due to being cut'; 'problems with tear in vagina'; and 'sore episiotomy scar'. Two-thirds (36) of the women had consulted their doctors and 12 had been referred for specialist opinion and/or treatment.

Only one of the women reporting perineal problems had delivered by Caesarean section, much less than the 16.4% section rate in the sample as a whole; and a forceps delivery was more frequent (52%) than among all vaginal deliveries (23.5%). The forceps association was present equally in primiparae and multiparae. All but one of the vaginal deliveries with this class of complaint had either an episiotomy (39) or a perineal tear (11) or both (1). This 75%

episiotomy rate was much greater than the 52% among all vaginal deliveries. Among 284 women having a pudendal nerve block, 6 (2.4%) reported later perineal symptoms, a statistically significant excess.

Discriminant analyses of these perineal problems confirmed that forceps delivery and pudendal block were positive predictors and Caesarean section a negative one. Episiotomy was not an independent predictor, forceps taking precedence. Among these 53 women, 13 (24.5%) also reported stress incontinence, which is greater than the sample mean, but only two (3.8%) reported urinary frequency.

We now regret not including perineal problems within our list of specific questions. Many women probably regard perineal symptoms as commonplace and fail to report them unless specifically asked.

Paraesthesias – numbness or tingling in the hands, fingers, feet and toes were the subjects of specific questions. Other paraesthesias were reported under the open question by an additional 37 women. They included 8 women with numbness around their Caesarean section scar; 2 with facial (Bell's) palsies; one with carpal tunnel syndrome; 4 with loss of sensation (rather than tingling) in the toes or lower leg; and 22 with numbness and/or tingling in the back, buttocks or thighs. The medical consultation rate for this category was low: 14 (38%) of the 37 had gone to the doctor, and only 3 were referred. Six women reported short duration symptoms (six weeks to six months) but 19 (51%) said they still had symptoms at the time of our enquiry.

Seven (32%) of the 22 women with back/buttocks/upper leg symptoms had had a Caesarean section, compared with 16% among the total population, and 7 (32%) had a forceps delivery. A procedural delivery was twice as frequent (64%) as in the whole sample. In addition, all but 2 of these 22 women (91%) had had epidural anaesthesia. Nine of them (41%) also had backache. Three out of the 4 with numbness in the lower leg had had an epidural; and 7 of the 8 with section-scar numbness; also one of the two facial palsies. If we set aside the section scars, the facial palsies and the carpal tunnel syndrome, which suggest other special mechanisms, the relative risk of these paraesthesias among epidural deliveries was 12.0.

Discriminant analysis confirmed epidural anaesthesia as the dominant predictive factor. Not surprisingly, since several women had section scar numbness, Caesarean section was the other significant predictive factor.

Long-term paraesthesias in the back, buttocks and legs look on this evidence as though they might represent an additional, although very low-frequency (0.48%), result of epidural anaesthesia. It is one that the enquiry would have missed had we not included the open question, however because an epidural induces numbness when it is in place, women with epidurals might selectively report any later numbness, having attributed it to the epidural. The relationship should therefore be subjected to specific enquiry in further investigations. It is known that similar paraesthesias occasionally occur as short-term effects following epidural anaesthesia. (Crawford, 1985b)

Mood disturbances additional to those already listed under 'depression and anxiety' were reported by 36 women. Seven reported a loss of interest in sex and the remaining 29 women reported a wide variety of disturbances, including inability to concentrate: feelings of alienation: nightmares: mild agoraphobia: and guilt feelings. Only 13 (36%) of these women had consulted a doctor, although 19 (53%) still had the symptom at the time of questioning. Two of the 13 (15%) who went to their doctors were referred for specialist consultation and/or treatment. Of the 7 women reporting loss of interest in sex, only one had consulted a doctor, even though for 5 of them the problem continued.

Fourteen (39%) of these 36 women had already reported depression/anxiety and 22 (61%) had reported extreme tiredness. Six (17%) had reported frequent headaches. We found no associations on simple discriminant analysis, with any obstetric, anaesthetic or maternal characteristics, apart from primiparity.

Thrush and other genital infections presenting as new symptoms within three months of the delivery, and lasting for more than six weeks were reported by 32 women. They are in themselves common complaints, and probably experienced by many other women who did not report them. However symptoms lasting more than six weeks are less common, and a spontaneous response to an open question might indicate especially troublesome symptoms. In fact 30 (94%) of the women had been to their doctor and 5 were referred for specialist consultation. Eighteen (56%) of the 32 complaints were unresolved at the time of our enquiry. These infections were not related to any of the obstetric or anaesthetic factors and the only apparent excess, confirmed by discriminant analysis, was among women under twenty-five years.

Prolapse and related symptoms were reported by 26 women, including 5 women with problems of faecal control. Eighteen of the 26 (69%) had consulted their doctors and 9 were referred for specialist advice and subsequent treatment (usually surgery).

All but one of these 26 women had had a vaginal delivery and among them 48% had forceps compared with 23.5% among all vaginal deliveries. Second stage labour of more than an hour occurred in 40%, compared with 29%; and only one women out of the 25 had an intact perineum, the remainder having an episiotomy or a laceration. Discriminant analyses nominated forceps and a long second stage as the primary predictors, while episiotomy and laceration were submerged by these dominating events. Not surprisingly, many of these same women had also reported bladder problems: 14 (54%) had stress incontinence, and 8 (31%) had urinary frequency.

The open question elicited many other symptoms and conditions apart from those described above: the 137 complaints falling within 60-70 different groups, each experienced by one, or two or three women.

Discussion

This chapter describes responses to several different questions directed to several different purposes. Some of them were deliberately ill-defined, and designed as much to control the overall quality of the reports analysed in earlier chapters, as to supplement the overall morbidity picture. Some of the specific questions amounted to oblique tests of reporting style, especially of over-reporting and neuroticism. These uses will be described in the next chapter. The open-ended question was also designed in part to supplement this approach, but mainly to complement the morbidity picture. In the event, the open question raised a number of issues demanding more specific questioning on future studies.

Several points of general or special interest emerged. Varicose veins were not associated with any delivery factors. This was not of great intrinsic interest especially since varicose veins generally start before delivery, but the negative finding provided indirect validation of the detected obstetric predictors of other symptoms. It helps dispel any suspicion that earlier results might arise from procedure-induced reporting biases.

The question on high blood pressure was designed to illuminate the subsequent natural history of gestational hypertension and pre-eclampsia: how often and for how long does hypertension in these categories continue after delivery? The responses seemed to show that hypertension continued for at least six weeks – usually for much longer than this – in about 8% of cases. This, at least, was the understanding of the women, and it seemed also to represent the views of the general practitioners as asserted by the treatment they supplied. There was no distinction between cases having proteinuric hypertension and labelled as pre-eclampsia, or as straightforward gestational hypertension. The scientific literature on the rate and duration of continuing hypertension is sketchy. The issue requires direct investigation, including medical validation.

Questions on general gastro-intestinal symptoms, expressed as 'bowel upsets' and 'indigestion', as well as dental problems, were included initially to control responses to other questions, particularly in relation to epidural anaesthesia. They showed no association with this procedure. However, 'bowel upsets' were interpreted by some women to include haemorrhoids, and perhaps also problems of faecal control. This was then reflected in a pattern of common associations with long second stage labour and forceps delivery.

The 'neurological' symptoms of buzzing in the ears, visual disturbances and dizziness or fainting were all increased after a general and spinal anaesthesia and pethidine was associated with visual disturbances. There were also relationships between the last two symptoms and epidural anaesthesia but the visual disturbance association was probably indirect, effected through cross-relationships between these symptoms and migraine. The open-ended question did however reveal one additional rare likely consequence of epidural anaesthesia: a pattern of sensation-loss and tingling in the back, buttocks, thighs and lower leg. The frequency was very low but the relative risk was high, and the association almost specific. Kitzinger's (1987) self-selected group of women who had epidurals (see Chapter 8) also described tingling or numbness in the lower back or legs, as a long-term side effect. She does not give the proportion reporting this nor its duration. No information is available either from Kitzinger's work or from our own on the severity of this complaint, but it merits further enquiry.

Chapter 15 – Symptom-Clusters and 'Syndromes'

We have concentrated up to now upon relationships between independent and dependent variables. By independent variables we generally mean those recorded in the case notes, including the social factors, the events and circumstances of delivery, and particular obstetric and anaesthetic procedures. A few were recorded immediately after the delivery, for example birthweight, infant length, and head circumference. The dependent variables were the symptoms recorded in the questionnaire by the mother herself, thirteen months to nine years later.

For most purposes the distinction was serviceable and reasonably clear-cut. We then relied upon a combination of detailed tabulations and discriminant analyses to identify the separate relationships of the different social and obstetric variables, even though they were themselves correlated with each other. We used the relative strengths and consistencies of their individual relationships with different dependent variables, and the mutually standardised measures of association obtained through discriminant analyses, to identify potential cause-effect relationships. We could thus judge which of the dependent variables (i.e. symptoms) could plausibly be regarded as potential consequences of particular antecedent factors; and which of them could be regarded as the principal and subsidiary components of groups of symptoms, or 'syndromes'.

However in order to ensure that health problems could potentially have their origins in the events of a particular birth, we always had to exclude recurrences or continuations of symptoms and in the interests of validity we discarded all inadequately recorded symptoms. The need to exclude certain reported symptoms created a methodological problem. If the reasons for excluding or including the response to a particular question were correlated with the reasons for excluding or including another – for example careless completion or a fickle memory – then this would create false correlations between the responses which were included. At the extremes, some women would record nothing reliably, and others would report many symptoms. In addition, some symptoms might reflect pre-existing states – for example pain tolerance variations – which themselves would influence the responses to other questions: as well as, possibly, the events of the delivery.

We tried to circumvent some of these issues by occasionally using one symptom for standardisation – treating it as a confounder – while testing the dependence of another upon delivery factors. We could thus show whether the obstetric and/or anaesthetic predictors of the symptom of interest, were equally powerful when the predictive power of the second symptom had been taken into account.

However, and apart from identifying a few notable overlaps, we have not looked systematically for different 'syndromes' or symptom-groups. Where we have postulated the existence of syndromes we have relied chiefly upon demonstrations of common sets of social or obstetric predictors, together with external knowledge and external models. Such models were drawn, for example, from neuro-anatomical connections (the neck and the arm) and known procedural groups (general anaesthesia used for Caesarean section). In this chapter, by contrast, we look at symptom-clustering as a primary phenomenon, without relying upon such guidance.

Technical causes of symptom-aggregation

We commented in Chapter 7 on the numbers of women who had none, one, two... different symptoms (Table 7.4). Symptoms were 'acceptable' for analysis as potential long term consequences of childbirth if they started within three months, lasted more than six weeks and were new. All such symptoms occurred in 47% of the population: and 12.5% of the population recorded three or more symptoms. This did not in itself indicate the presence or absence of a tendency for symptoms to 'aggregate', but the data now presented in Table 15.1 show evident variation in the numbers of *additional* symptoms which accompanied each specific symptom. Thus, 29% of women with backache and 32% of women with stress incontinence complained of that symptom alone and no others: but only 6% of those with pain in the arms or weakness in the arms. Conversely, over 40% of women with pain in the arms or weakness in the arms or weakness in the legs, reported five or more additional symptoms: compared with only 7% of those with stress incontinence or haemorrhoids.

We also constructed matrices of association between each symptom and each other symptom (see later) which confirmed the existence of many separate and sometimes quite localised, pairs of correlated symptoms; and sometimes of larger groups. However, there was in addition a widespread and pervasive background of less powerful cross-associations; at this lower level, almost everything was correlated with everything else. Much of this could be attributed to the technicalities of the data-acquisition and 'acceptance' processes, as briefly outlined above.

Selective reporting artefacts occurred at several different levels. Not every women received a questionnaire; and not all of those believed to have received one, filled it in and replied. There is a possibility of some element of bias at both levels. At the first level there were social differences in migration. At the second

TABLE 15.1

Extent to which each symptom was accompanied by other symptoms

Number (%) of women reporting:

	Just that symptom	Additional symptoms 1	Additional symptoms 2 – 4	Additional symptoms 5+	Total women
Frequent headaches	65 (16)	67 (16)	196 (47)	91 (22)	419
Neckache	18 (8)	29 (13)	103 (45)	78 (34)	228
Shoulderache	20 (8)	56 (21)	114 (43)	73 (28)	263
Backache	477 (29)	428 (26)	563 (34)	166 (10)	1634
Pain in arms	7 (6)	13 (12)	41 (38)	47 (44)	108
Pain in legs	42 (17)	55 (23)	71 (30)	72 (30)	240
Weak arms	9 (6)	18 (13)	54 (38)	61 (43)	142
Weak legs	12 (8)	20 (14)	51 (34)	65 (44)	148
Bowel upset	52 (16)	82 (26)	121 (38)	66 (21)	321
Tingling hands/fingers	44 (15)	56 (19)	126 (43)	67 (23)	293
Tingling feet/toes	12 (9)	14 (11)	55 (44)	45 (36)	126
Buzzing in ears	5 (7)	6 (5)	38 (50)	27 (36)	76
Flashing lights/spots	16 (9)	36 (21)	71 (41)	51 (29)	174
Dizzy/faint	22 (10)	36 (17)	91 (43)	62 (29)	211
Migraine	25 (15)	24 (15)	75 (45)	41 (25)	165
Indigestion	19 (15)	26 (20)	55 (43)	27 (21)	127
Urinary frequency	82 (12)	196 (29)	296 (44)	94 (14)	668
Stress incontinence	577 (32)	520 (29)	557 (31)	128 (7)	1782
High blood pressure	14 (29)	12 (25)	17 (35)	5 (10)	48
Piles	318 (34)	240 (26)	306 (33)	67 (7)	931
Varicose veins	37 (25)	47 (31)	47 (31)	20 (13)	151
Dental problems	31 (25)	28 (23)	46 (37)	19 (15)	124
Depression/anxiety	231 (22)	291 (27)	430 (40)	113 (11)	1065
Extreme tiredness	294 (21)	391 (27)	594 (42)	148 (10)	1427
Other	117 (28)	93 (22)	157 (37)	56 (13)	423

level women who had several symptoms are likely to be more motivated to reply than those who had one or none. The effect must amount to an extension of 'Berkson's fallacy', in which patients selected on the grounds of ill health – e.g. hospital admissions – tend to show false correlations between one illness and another. It was for this reason that we sought to demonstrate (Chapter 4) that the obstetric and anaesthetic characteristics (including parity) of responders did not differ in any major and relevant way from the total sample to whom the questionnaires were sent; and that we had in fact achieved a high overall *response* rate among those who received questionnaires – in contrast with the rather low *return* rate for the full enquiry.

The main technical source of the 'background level' of aggregation of symptoms was probably related to variations in the levels of accuracy and detail with which different women composed their replies. Some of this variation would arise from varying levels of motivation, some of it from variations in technical competence in understanding and answering questions, and some of it from variations in accuracy of recall. For example, we found some instances of apparent confusion between one pregnancy and another; the number of inadequately dated symptoms increased with greater parity (Table 15.2); and there were some possible confusions between antenatal and post-partum onsets. We have also shown in Chapter 4 that the accuracy of symptom recording varied over time, with more inadequately dated reports following the earlier deliveries. For whatever reason, a woman who reported one symptom to

TABLE 15.2

Number of inadequately dated symptoms according to parity

No. of inadequately dated symptoms	Parity 0 No. (% in group)	1 No. (% in group)	2 No. (% in group)	3 or more No. (% in group)
One	539 (12.9)	679 (14.5)	304 (15.4)	124 (14.3)
Two	208 (5.0)	321 (6.9)	140 (7.1)	69 (7.9)
Three	102 (2.4)	155 (3.3)	86 (4.3)	45 (5.2)
Four or more	140 (3.3)	204 (4.4)	145 (7.3)	82 (9.4)
Total women	4185	4669	1978	869

the levels of accuracy and detail which made it acceptable for our main analyses, would probably report others in like manner: while those who failed to reach the acceptance level for one symptom would probably do so for others as well. Levels of acceptance-selection differed for different symptoms (see Figure 7.1), and the likelihood of artefactual cross-correlations would also vary.

In addition to variations in the accuracy of reporting different symptoms, there was some overlap between the content of the different questions. For example, a woman with migraine might report her problems under 'frequent headache', 'flashing lights' and 'neckache' – and perhaps under 'migraine' as well. There was evidence that some women with haemorrhoids had interpreted this additionally as a 'bowel upset'; and that some women with widespread backache, who were not sure whether to report it as middle backache or lower backache, reported both.

Finally, certain subsets of the population seemed relatively prone to symptoms of particular broad classes. For example, Asian women complained more of spinal-axis and limb discomforts: this alone, – even in the absence of a genuine syndrome – would be sufficient to create a pattern of population-wide correlations between these symptoms. Likewise, older women had more stress incontinence, and this would be sufficient to create a pattern of correlation between this symptom and any other symptom (e.g. fatigue) which was also reported preferentially in this group of older women. Similarly, women who had delivered a baby quite recently reported more symptoms than those who had delivered some time ago, probably because they remembered more: and this in turn would create a pattern of aggregation between symptoms recorded or remembered preferentially on this basis.

We pursued these ideas by carrying out a discriminant analysis to try to 'predict' those women who reported one or more symptoms, compared with those reporting none; and we carried out another to identify the terms on which we could predict women who had four or more symptoms, compared with three or less. The results are given in Table 15.3. Many of the factors demonstrated in this Table have already been shown to be predictive of different specific symptoms: and of high-frequency symptoms in particular. Examples include the relationship between epidural anaesthesia and backache; greater birthweight and long second-stage labour with stress incontinence; forceps delivery and long second-stage labour with haemorrhoids; and a long first stage with extreme tiredness and depression. That is, the physical and objective facts of delivery remained as effective predictors; together with Asian ethnic group and primiparity. The latter is explicable partly in terms of its obstetric associations and partly in terms of reduced exclusions of recurrent symptoms. The factor most difficult to account for here was breast feeding. This had been a

TABLE 15.3

Discriminant analysis to predict number of symptoms reported

Vaginal deliveries
(1) One or more symptoms compared with none

Factor	F-value
Primiparity	33.494
Breast feeding	17.786
Forceps	13.008
Large birthweight	11.253
Long 2nd stage labour	11.003
Epidural	9.3814
Long 1st stage labour	6.1934
Pethidine	5.3407
No episiotomy	4.6429

(2) Four or more symptoms compared with three or less
(Women with no symptoms excluded)

Multiple delivery	9.1204
Asian race	8.8480
Long 1st stage labour	7.0269
Younger maternal age	6.1542

predictor of depression and extreme tiredness, but not of such magnitude as to account for its presence here.

All these inter-relationships together resulted in a complex matrix of cross-associations, probably containing both artefacts and genuine components, which might prove very difficult to dissect. And this indeed was how it turned out.

Identifying clusters

We tried two main methods of identifying clusters of symptoms. The first was a statistical 'cluster analysis' and the second was the construction of a matrix of cross-correlations, followed by informal and intuitive interpretation. Formal cluster analysis turned out to be exceedingly expensive of computer time and space and, in practical terms, demanded repeated sub-analyses of limited subsets of the whole material. Initial examinations along these lines showed up only the clusters of which we were aleady aware, and we turned our attention instead to constructing a correlation matrix.

For the matrices of association between symptoms and social and obstetric variables, as demonstrated in earlier chapters the temporal direction of the relationship was always clear: since symptoms always followed the delivery. This allowed the use of the Relative Risk (RR) statistic: the ratio between the risks of a particular consequence in 'exposed' and 'non-exposed' groups. However, the relationships between separate post-delivery symptoms were not guided by any such prior constraint and the RR-statistic was not appropriate. Because of this, and because all the symptoms were binary variables – scaled as either 'yes' or 'no' – we related each symptom to every other through a matrix of 'Odds Ratios'. The Odds Ratio (OR) is also the ratio between two other ratios: in this case the yes:no ratio (Odds) for the second variable, when the first variable is present: and the similar ratio when the first variable is absent.

The OR statistic has the advantage of symmetry; the numerical value is the same whichever of the two variations is taken to be the 'first' or the 'second'. Where there is no association the OR is 1.0: when both tend to be present together, the OR is between 1.0 and infinity: and when one variable tends to be present in the absence of the other, the OR is between 0.0 and 1.0.

In fact, using the adequately dated and 'acceptable' symptoms included in our discriminant studies, all but two of the measured OR values were greater than 1.0. ie, positively associated. This provides a dramatic confirmation of the expectations (and the problems) outlined in previous paragraphs. The main problem, as it now appeared, was to identify the more striking OR values against this background, and to attempt an interpretation. Table 15.4 displays the distribution of OR values within the different ranges: the 300 calculations in each column represent all the possible pairs of symptoms among the listed 25. This table compares three different distributions: (1) all symptoms included as 'acceptable' in our main analysis of predictors; (2) those which were reported following delivery but inadequately recorded and (3) the full set of unselected reports: i.e. every symptom occurring after delivery irrespective of onset, duration, previous presence or adequate dating. This confirms the extent to which selection in terms of quality of recording, results in a 'background' of artefactual aggregation, compared with the full unselected data-set.

TABLE 15.4

Odds-Ratio distribution
300 symptom-pairs from 25 symptoms

OR	n_1	n_2	n_3
0 -2.5	76	10	160
-5.0	107	98	107
-7.5	45	88	18
-10.0	24	35	7
-12.5	16	23	4
-15.0	8	9	–
-17.5	4	9	–
-20.0	4	5	–
-25.0	6	7	1
-30.0	4	6	2
-35.0	2	3	1
>35.0	4	7	–
	300	300	300

n_1 – are Odds Ratios for frequencies of symptoms meeting the 'acceptance' criteria for inclusion in main analysis of determinants

n_2 – are Odds Ratios for the inadequately recorded symptoms

n_3 – are Odds Ratios for all reported symptoms occurring after delivery, irrespective of onset, duration, previous history, or adequate dating

TABLE 15.5

Stress incontinence and urinary frequency

		Stress incontinence		
		No	Yes	Totals
Urinary	No	9667	1366	11033
Frequency	Yes	252	416	668
	Totals	9919	1782	11701

$$RR = 11.68$$
$$X^2 (1) = 1210.7$$

For the symptoms falling within our 'acceptance-criteria', odds-ratios up to about 5.0 were commonplace and could not be distinguished reliably from the presumably artefactual 'background' level. But higher values deserve more detailed study. The following synopses are based upon selecting those groups whose mutual odds-ratios stand out as discrete islands against this background.

Perineal symptoms

As shown in Table 15.5, stress incontinence and urinary frequency tended to occur together. The OR was 11.7. For each separately, and for both jointly, these two symptoms were relatively isolated from all others except themselves. Apart from urinary frequency, the most powerful association of stress incontinence was with 'bowel upsets' (OR = 3.1). As the open-ended question sometimes indicated (see Chapter 14), this may reflect the occasional co-occurrence of faecal incontinence. Neither of these bladder symptoms was strongly associated with haemorrhoids (OR = 2.4 for incontinence; 2.2 for frequency), despite their common associations with pelvic trauma. We have already interpreted this to indicate that the physical mechanisms of the injuries probably differed. Haemorrhoids themselves were not strongly associated with anything else: the strongest were with varicose veins (OR = 4.2) and bowel upsets (OR = 3.2): the first is probably an indication of common susceptibilities, and the second probably represents a double statement of the same symptom. Neither of the two bladder symptoms was strongly associated with fatigue or with depression or with backache, and the most powerful external association of urinary frequency was with weakness in the legs (OR = 4.5).

The two bladder symptoms together therefore constitute a small and distinctive island of aggregation, clearly visible against the general background of 'technical' aggregation. And – as shown earlier – both stress incontinence reported singly, and urinary frequency combined with stress incontinence, showed clear associations with prolonged and traumatic deliveries. This is compatible with earlier evidence that the principal forms of injury related to stress incontinence, with or without accompanying urinary frequency are distinctive, probably occurring through direct muscular damage or neural compression: and the mechanisms probably differ from the mechanisms responsible for urinary frequency in the absence of stress incontinence, or for haemorrhoids.

Depression and fatigue

Anxiety/depression and extreme tiredness exhibited a strong mutual correlation (OR = 9.1), again standing well clear of the general background of technical aggregation. There were no strong associations with the other frequently reported symptoms including bladder symptoms, haemorrhoids backache, headache, and migraine. In particular, there was no strong association with headache/migraine unassociated with backache, even though this shared common social predictors with depression. Nor were there any strong associations with the vaguely defined gastro-intestinal symptoms which had been included chiefly as controls against the promiscuous reporting of symptoms in general. Neither depression/anxiety nor extreme tiredness were among those symptoms (Table 15.1) presenting with high rates of multiple problems; they were 7th and 8th, respectively, among the list of symptoms which were accompanied by no other complaints; and even where they did not occur alone they often combined with only one other symptom. The strongest of the external associations for depression and fatigue were with weakness in the arms (OR = 3.3 and 5.1), weakness in the legs (OR = 4.1 and 6.0), visual disturbances (OR = 3.5 and 5.3), dizziness/fainting (OR = 4.8 and 5.0) and buzzing in the ears (OR = 4.4 and 3.4) The first two of these symptoms can probably be regarded as double reporting of general severe fatigue; the others might indicate a common element of 'neuroticism'.

These findings confirm the inferences drawn from the similar patterns of predictors of depression and of fatigue. They were broadly alike, except for maternal age, and the additional fatigue associations with post-partum haemorrhage and nitrous oxide, as demonstrated in Chapter 13. We might suppose that some of the differentiation between depression and fatigue was a question of the manner in which they were 'labelled': but there is also a mechanistic reason for the association. Fatigue, lassitude and insomnia are recognised symptoms of depression: while sleeplessness, 'overload' and fatigue are among the precipitating causes of depression.

Frequent Headaches and Migraine

Reports of frequent headache were strongly correlated with reports of migraine (OR = 25.0), and there was evidence indicating a high level of double reporting (see Chapter 9). Both migraine and frequent headache were associated with visual disturbances (OR = 20.2 and 10.7), dizziness and fainting (OR = 12.1 and 12.0) and buzzing in the ears (OR = 17.2 and 12.3). Most of this fits well with our understanding of the established syndrome of migraine except for buzzing in the ears. This occurred only in a small number of cases, but is not a regular component of classical migraine, although there is a recognised uncommon form of the condition characterised by tinnitus and vertigo and believed to involve the vertebral and basilar arteries.

We wondered whether some cases of headache might have been triggered by an undetected dural injury. Overt spinal headache can indeed be accompanied by tinnitus and vertigo, (Wang et al 1987) and the headache is clearly related to posture, which might also be interpreted as 'dizziness'. However this remains no more than a tentative question and the answer is beyond the resolution of the present data set.

Unexpectedly, women reporting high blood pressure also reported buzzing in the ears (OR = 14.6). In this case, a simple explanation might be that the tinnitus became a cause of anxiety, that this took the patient to the doctor, and that the doctor then discovered – or perhaps mis-diagnosed – hypertension. Anyway the numbers affected here were small.

The cluster of headache and migraine and its associated symptoms were therefore reasonably consistent with the syndrome as it is generally understood, but sufficiently exceptional in points of detail to deserve further enquiry. There was one additional finding to add to this disquiet concerning its true nature, namely a high relative prevalence, among affected women, of pains and weaknesses in the arms and legs, and paraesthesias in the hands and feet. We return to this point later.

Backache and spinal-axis symptoms

Middle backache and lower backache were strongly associated with each other (OR = 10.5). Middle backache, a little more than lower backache, was also strongly associated with neckache and shoulderache (OR = 8.2 and 7.5). Apart from this fairly powerful correlation with pain in an adjacent anatomical site, the remaining associations of backache ranged only from moderate to weak. For example, middle backache was only moderately associated with headache and migraine (OR = 4.3, 4.6), and the associations of lower backache with these symptoms were weaker still. We have had to rely here chiefly upon their common obstetric correlates, to confirm that this is a genuine association.

There were rather stronger associations between middle backache and the limb symptoms including pains in the arms and legs (OR = 7.0 and 5.9), weakness in the arms and legs (OR = 7.2 and 8.8) and tingling/numbness in the hands and feet (OR = 4.8 and 5.6). The associations between lower backache and these same symptoms were weaker than those of middle backache, even for the leg symptoms. If it were not for the external evidence linking backache with neckache and headache, these findings could not be interpreted as evidence for the existence of a syndrome formulated in terms of anatomical adjacencies. We recall the similar inconsistencies (Chapter 10) between the postulated posturally-determined spinal-axis-syndrome, with its increased prevalence in Asian women, but where the details of the symptom-complexes tended to be aberrant in those same women. The patterns of association were not therefore as simple as was first supposed. We shall develop alternative postulates later.

Neck and shoulderache

There were strong associations between frequent headache and neckache (OR = 9.2), headache and shoulderache (OR = 5.9), and shoulderache and neckache (OR = 9.2). This constellation of symptoms, at the upper end of the spinal axis, seemed set apart from the (earlier) pattern of spinal-axis symptoms radiating from the back. This seems to indicate an additional overlapping syndrome, and this hypothesis is supported through the common cross-associations of these symptoms with general anaesthesia and Caesarean section, although relatively small numbers of women were affected. However, there were several additional and sometimes anatomically remote associations with lower as well as upper limb-symptoms, which again suggested that the pattern of relationships was more complex than it first appeared. This raises issues comparable with those noted in the previous paragraph.

Gastro-intestinal symptoms

These vaguely defined and more trivial symptoms – 'bowel upsets', 'indigestion' and 'dental problems' – were included chiefly as control variables. It is appropriate to consider them at this point. We included them in order to seek contrasts between them, and other symptoms, in the strengths of their respective associations with obstetric and anaesthetic events: and particularly with respect to epidural anaesthesia. We hoped also to test the independence of associations between obstetric procedures and genuine problems, from any tendencies towards general over-reporting. If there were a sub-section of the population which did tend to over-report, then this might have been manifest in cross-correlations between different symptoms within this less definable and minor group. It might have shown also as cross-association with such complaints as buzzing in the ears, visual disturbances, dizziness and fainting, frequent headaches, weaknesses and fatigue, and peripheral paraesthesias. As it happened, these other complaints fell within separately definable groups with sufficient consistency to suggest that most of them were genuine physical symptoms: although this is not to say that some of them might not be the symptoms of anxiety neurosis. The 'dummy' intestinal questions and dental problems showed very few interactions with depression or with fatigue: or indeed with any other of the frequently reported problems.

Among the dental/intestinal symptoms themselves, the most powerful interaction was between indigestion and dental problems (OR = 5.7). For indigestion the greatest external associations were with migraine (OR = 7.8), and with the other symptoms related to migraine. A report of 'indigestion' in these circumstances may simply be an indicator of the nausea which goes with migraine.

Other external associations of these intestinal problems were more enigmatic. There were associations between the dental problems and both varicose veins (OR = 7.1) and buzzing in the ears (OR = 6.8). Both are difficult to interpret, although the explanation might lie in a common co-variation with increasing age. Varicose veins also exhibited an association with buzzing in the ears (OR = 5.5). For bowel upsets, the strongest associations were with tingling in the feet (OR = 9.4): with pain and weakness in the legs (OR = 8.0 and 8.1); and with buzzing in the ears (OR = 8.3).

In general, although these vague and trivial complaints showed some associations indicating an element of neuroticism, the lack of association with depression/anxiety, or with fatigue or the other high frequency symptoms suggests that neurotic or hypochondriacal responses were not a serious problem from the point of view of interpreting our other results.

Limb symptoms

Complaints of pain and weakness in the arms and in the legs, and paraesthesias in the hands and feet, displayed an extraordinary concentration of cross correlations. The matrix of odds-ratios for all possible pairings, together with neckache and shoulderache, is given in Table 15.6. We have already noted the strength of the overlap between neckache and shoulderache, but there are several other odds ratios in this Table which are just as striking: some even more so. There were associations between different symptoms in the same limb, and between the same symptom in different limbs. There were major interactions between pain and weakness in the arm: between paraesthesias in the hands and paraesthesias in the feet: between pain and weakness in the legs: and between weakness in the arms and in the legs. Whatever its explanation, physical or emotional, it can scarcely be ignored. The levels of association are far beyond those attributable to 'technical background', and they do not seem to represent simply double reporting of vaguely identified symptoms. For example, there was no systematic correspondence within the separate anatomical contiguities. A search for a localised anatomical injury would have to consider the possibility of vascular embarrassment or other injury of the cervical spinal cord. It would seem far more likely that these symptom-clusters represent either an emotional disorder or a non-focal pathological disorder.

TABLE 15.6

Matrix of odds ratios: limb girdle and limb symptoms

Symptom		(2)	(3)	(4)	(5)	(6)	(7)	(8)
Neckache	(1)	90.2	22.1	16.9	11.5	7.4	10.8	11.0
Shoulderache	(2)	x	20.7	15.6	7.4	7.8	9.7	8.8
Pain in arms	(3)	–	x	84.7	27.5	35.5	23.3	24.6
Weakness in arms	(4)	–	–	x	19.6	18.9	99.3	17.7
Paraesthesia in hands/fingers	(5)	–	–	–	x	7.1	9.0	85.9
Pain in legs	(6)	–	–	–	–	x	32.7	14.5
Weakness in legs	(7)	–	–	–	–	–	x	27.3
Paraesthesia in feet/toes	(8)	–	–	–	–	–	–	x

As we noted earlier, these limb symptoms showed strong associations with reports of migraine and of buzzing in the ears, visual disturbances and dizziness/fainting. There were additional correlations with 'bowel upsets' and varicose veins. For these reasons we have to consider the possibility that this concentration of symptoms might be a manifestation of 'neurotic tendencies' and that women who believe rather vaguely that they have something wrong with them, tend to over-report this particular constellation of symptoms. However, the localisation and strength of this pattern of limb cross-correlations (Table 15.6) is sufficiently remarkable, and displays sufficiently striking exceptions, as to cast doubt upon this hypothesis: at least as a major explanation. In particular, as Table 15.7 shows, the pattern of associations did not extend to the pelvic-perineal symptoms, or to reports of depressive illness or of extreme tiredness.

A major clue to the nature of this group of symptoms – with its failure to reflect anatomical contiguities and adjacencies – is the extraordinarily high prevalence of most of the components among Asian women. This suggests that at least part of this symptom-complex represents the bone tenderness and muscle-weakness of osteomalacia. Some accounts of osteomalacia mention involvement of the audiotory ossicles and this might provide a partial explanation of the correlations with tinnitus and vertigo; tinnitus was also more frequent among Asian women although numbers were very small. The associations between these symptoms, displayed as Odds Ratios, are set out in Table 15.7.

TABLE 15.7

Limb, neck and shoulder symptoms v migraine-type symptoms

Matrix of Odds Ratios

	Neckache	Shoulder	Arms Pain	Arms Weakness	Tingling in hands	Legs Pain	Legs Weakness	Tingling in feet
Headache	9.2	5.9	6.8	6.4	5.8	6.0	6.4	5.3
Migraine	4.9	4.6	10.3	9.0	5.3	8.4	9.3	7.9
Buzzing in ears	12.3	6.1	13.6	10.1	14.9	10.4	14.2	16.9
Visual disturbance	10.7	9.8	12.6	10.6	6.7	7.1	12.3	3.2
Fainting/dizziness	7.9	5.7	13.6	12.4	8.3	8.4	13.1	10.5
Lower backache	4.1	3.9	4.4	4.5	2.5	4.8	5.1	5.2
Bowel upsets	3.6	3.0	8.0	8.1	4.5	5.0	6.9	9.4
Stress incontinence	2.1	1.5	2.0	1.5	2.0	1.7	1.4	1.8
Urinary frequency	3.1	2.5	2.7	3.6	2.3	2.4	4.5	3.4
Haemorrhoids	1.8	1.6	1.3	1.7	1.2	1.9	2.0	1.7
Depression	3.3	3.2	3.6	3.3	2.1	2.7	4.1	2.9
Tiredness	4.5	4.0	4.5	5.1	3.4	2.6	6.0	3.4

This osteomalacia hypothesis will require direct verification but, even in its formative stages, it seems to provide an important key to interpretation, providing a central element within a generalised model of the pathogenesis of several components of post-partum morbidity for the Asian women. But it may not be limited to the Asian women. We shall discuss the structure of a more general explanatory model in the next chapter.

Inverse prediction

At this point we tried to clarify the situation by seeing whether we could predict particular obstetric events and procedures in reverse, on the basis of subsequently reported symptoms. For this examination, the 'dependent' variables – the symptoms recorded in the questionnaire – were used to distinguish between women 'exposed' and 'not exposed' to earlier social. obstetric and anaesthetic circumstances and occurrences. We did however incorporate age and parity as important additional confounders within these analyses and we made comparisons which included all ethnic groups, and others limited to Caucasians.

In general, however, these inverse examinations were less helpful than we had hoped and added no more than a technical confirmation of earlier findings based on forward looking discrimination.

Conclusions

The independent variables – the social, obstetric and anaesthetic factors – together with all their cross-correlations were described in Chapter 6. The chapters following described the ways in which these factors predicted the various reported symptoms. In the present chapter we have completed a third set of cross-associations – those which describe the ways in which the different health problems relate to each other.

We have shown that our strict criteria for symptom acceptance together with other methodological technicalities, themselves resulted in a degree of mutual correlation between symptoms. On top of this there was some evidence of an element of multiple symptom reporting, that might be related to neurotic or hypochondriacal reactions, although this did not seem to be extensive. However, the main explanations of the major symptom-clusters and cross-associations more probably related to the several different underlying postulated mechanisms of causation identified within the data set, each of them shared by particular symptom groups.

Chapter 16 – Synthesis

In this chapter we draw together the main findings of the previous ones. The essential results of these enquiries were 1) the reporting of a large amount of self-perceived morbidity, specifically related to childbirth, and much of it chronic: and 2) the identification of numerous potential social and obstetric determinants, each related to its own specific components of this subsequent ill health.

These proposed determinants were located both within the social background and within the delivery process. However it was also possible to infer the presence of others within the previous obstetric history and within the post-partum environment. These relationships were embedded within a comprehensive matrix of associated events, some of them almost certainly representing cause-effect mechanisms, while other potential determinants were much more tentative. Some existed in relative isolation from others, but some were parts of complex and sometimes additive sequences and interactions.

We found it surprising, in view of the size and importance of the problem, that longer term post-partum morbidity seems never previously to have been documented in a systematic way. This comment applies equally to the measurements of prevalence and to the identification of possible causes. There have been one or two studies following-up specific problems, such as deep-vein thrombosis (Bergqvist et al 1990) or fertility after Caesarean (Hemminki, 1986), but none of a more widespread nature. For most of the conditions – with the exception of postnatal depression and stress incontinence – the literature was almost empty. Some conditions, such as backache or haemorrhoids, were known to occur in pregnancy or shortly after but neither the proportions of women affected nor the duration of the symptoms were known. Some conditions lacked more than a mention in the scientific literature or in standard text books: and some lacked even that. (eg Clayton et al, 1985; Hibbard, 1988; Iffy-Kaminetzky, 1981; Llewellyn-Jones 1990; Knor 1987).

We therefore hope and expect that our findings will stimulate a major endeavour in applied research and that this in turn will lead to major preventive and therapeutic programmes in several different areas. This might extend to such areas as nutritional policy, health education, antenatal care programmes, the refinement of particular procedures, an improved definition of their indications and contra-indications, and a redesign of the arrangements for post-partum surveillance.

In this chapter we review and collate our findings under three main headings. First, we review the overall prevalences of health problems among the women of the sample: and from this we extrapolate the findings to the population at large.

We indicate the scale of the burden of ill-health borne by the women, and the health-care loads borne by Health Services. Second, we review the ways in which our survey methods and analytical processes were developed against the needs of this particular enquiry; and this with a view to assisting in the design of others. Third we construct a model framework against which the findings can be interpreted: and against which fresh questions can be posed and new research designed. In the next chapter, and stepping tentatively beyond the results which this additional research may reveal, we speculate on the medium-term and long-term actions which should be planned, and the immediate action which should now be undertaken.

Prevalences: social and health care loads

Implications for women

In this population of 11701 post-partum women, just under half (47%) reported at least one symptom within three months of the delivery of the child, which continued for more than six weeks and which had never been experienced before. The total number reported was 11,645: a mean of 1:0 per woman. Some women reported no symptoms and others more than one. In England and Wales, with approximately 680,000 deliveries annually (1987), this would amount to 680,000 post-partum health problems (as defined above) experienced by around 320,000 parturient women.

Our research suggests that the majority of these symptoms were long-lasting, with as many as two-thirds (varying according to the specific problem) still continuing at the time of our investigation. The follow-up period ranged from thirteen months to nine years after the birth of the child, so that for many women these symptoms had become chronic. National extrapolation suggests that around 210,000 women each year develop about 450,000 post-delivery symptoms which are unlikely to resolve. These numbers, we recall, are for new symptoms; and if we had included recurrences, they would be higher. We should also recall that these estimates do not include incompletely dated symptoms and so must be regarded as minima. The cumulative prevalence of chronic health problems in women completing their families is difficult to estimate exactly, but it represents a very considerable burden. If women are exposed to accumulating risks of chronic complaints of this order with each successive baby, then a majority must eventually be affected. Childbirth must be far and away the major cause of chronic health problems among women in their child-rearing years.

The extrapolation of symptom prevalences from our sample to the general population are only approximate. In Chapter 6 we compared the sample with the national population of parturient women and found some differences. In particular the sample contained more older women, fewer in social classes IV and V, and Asian women who were socially atypical of their ethnic group. In addition there were more Caesarean sections and forceps deliveries and more epidurals administered. However some of these factors were positively, and others negatively, related to symptom-occurrence so that they were often counter-balanced. For example the sample excess of forceps deliveries with longer second stages would inflate the extrapolated prevalences of pelvic symptoms; but the more frequent Caesarean sections would concomitantly reduce them. The epidural associated spinal-axis symptoms in our sample might be more frequent than we would expect nationally, but elective sections, of which our sample had more, would counter-balance this to some extent. And the Asian women in the sample were of higher social class and lower parity than is usual for this group, so that we might expect sample based estimates of spinal-axis and limb symptoms, if they are related to nutritional deficiencies to be lower than in the general population. The social predictors of headache, depression and fatigue (e.g. unmarried status; lower social class) were under-represented in our sample; although the excess of older women in the sample might counter-balance this – at least for fatigue. Although the detailed prevalence-estimates for individual symptoms might vary a little from those in the general population it would seem that our overall estimates of post-partum morbidity give an adequate assessment for extrapolation to the wider scene.

We must not assume that every class of symptom which is demonstrably relatable to the events and circumstances surrounding delivery, is 'caused' physically by the events themselves. Some may be 'caused' by lifestyle changes following on from these events – for example the load of caring for twins; or the carrying and bending involved in child-care – and some of the individual symptoms within a heterogeneous group might have been entirely unrelated to childbirth or childcare. Conversely, however, many of the symptoms excluded because they were recurrences or continuations should probably not have been; some must have recurred or have been exacerbated through the events of childbirth. Some of those complaints without accurate dates attached to them were also probably related.

Our research-design did not include a 'control' group of women who had not had a child. In practice, we could not have obtained an acceptable control group with which to compare symptom frequencies, since most women have children, and those who are childless differ in so many other ways. For the purposes of identifying the potential determinants of symptoms we had no need for a separate external control group; the method was based upon internal comparisons.

For some purposes it might have seemed better to restrict our attention to symptoms starting within a week of delivery, rather than the first three months.

For many symptoms these did in fact constitute the majority. However, the distribution of symptom onsets within this wider period – and indeed within the whole of the first year – often provided valuable additional insights: insights which a prior narrow restriction would have masked. For some symptoms (e.g. haemorrhoids), those occurring after the first week were clearly not related to any delivery factors, while those occurring in the first week were. By contrast, other symptoms (e.g. backache) were still related to aspects of delivery, even when they started up to three months after the birth. Sometimes there were obvious combinations of potential determinants (as with headache or extreme fatigue), some of which were delivery-related and some childcare-related. A more restricted temporal acceptance-criterion would have hampered the separate identification of these relationships.

Whatever the specific 'causes' and whatever the criteria used to establish the connection between a symptom and its antecedents, it is clear that long-term post-partum morbidity is widespread. We know that many new symptoms lasted years, with a third of the sample reporting at least one that was still present at the time of the enquiry. The main residual gap in our knowledge about symptoms – on which our own study offers little – is an assessment of the severity of these health problems, and their impacts upon the lives of the affected women.

Implications for the Health Services

Much of the morbidity reported after childbirth was not reported to doctors. We do not know exactly why this should be so. We found little previous work on this issue in the scientific literature and we did not ourselves seek information on this point. Only for stress incontinence, which showed a particularly low rate of medical consultation, was there earlier reported work (Jolleys 1988). This was within a general female population, not a post-childbirth population. Here, too, very low consultation rates were found. When the women were asked why they had not consulted their doctor, 68% said that they did not consider this symptom to be a serious problem: 25% said the symptoms were too infrequent to warrant treatment, while 20% felt that it was just a usual female problem.

Whatever the stated and the true reasons for this reluctance to consult doctors might be, it had one clear effect. The extent and nature of long-term morbidity following childbirth has not been recognised by the medical profession at large (Hall, 1991). It is scarcely reported at all in the medical literature, and inadequately mentioned in the textbooks.

If the proportion of symptomatic women consulting their doctors was small, then the proportion referred for specialist consultation was smaller still. In our own sample, around 34% of all symptoms (3928) were taken to a doctor. But only 640 were referred. This represents around 5% of the symptoms reported in the questionnaires.

These consultation figures can also be extrapolated to the United Kingdom as a whole. Each year at least 330,000 women must seek at least one consultation with their general practitioner for one of their post-partum symptoms. The proportion of specialist referrals in our sample could be extrapolated to about 34,000 in the country as a whole each year. These figures refer only to 'first time' symptoms beginning within three months of delivery and lasting for more than six weeks. If we were to include consultations for short-term illnesses, recurrent or continuing symptoms, and symptoms whose exact specifications were not supplied to us – as well as repeat consultations for the same problem – the estimate of the load would be much greater.

Methods

In this section we review three main technical themes. The first is about the sampling methods employed, about the statistical reliability of results, about selection-bias and reporting-bias: and about the technical problems of extrapolating the findings to a wider context. The second is a retrospective look at the use of postal questionnaires, the possible hazards entailed, and the counter-balancing virtues of linking the results with existing medical records. The third is a reconsideration of the use of contingency tables, and especially of formal multivariate analysis, in order to pursue a crucial sequential argument, which begins by demonstrating a wide range of statistical associations, proceeds to identify primary associations and to separate them from secondary ones and finally attempts to identify potential determinants.

Sampling

The sample structure was opportunistic. The original objectives of the study related to the possible long-term effects of epidural anaesthesia. The proposal was formulated initially in the context which generated the question: a hospital specialising in the development of this technique. Although the scope of the investigation then widened (Chapter 1) it retained its original base; and its retention was reinforced by the existence of full computer-coded maternity records, with which the follow-up data could later be linked.

Birmingham in general has a higher proportion of births to Asian and Afro-Caribbean women (Chapter 6), but the location of the hospital within the city resulted in a reduced representation compared with the total city population. Fortuitously, this was close to the national picture. However, the Asian women in the hospital sample were socially atypical of Asian women living in Birmingham: and presumably in the country as a whole. Their social class and parity distributions were closer to that of the Caucasians.

As we have already noted, follow-up was hampered by the high rate of migration in the period (up to nine years) since the children were born, and this was hindered further by the refusal of the Local Medical Committee to sanction the use of the Family Practitioner Committee (now Family Health Service Authority) register in order to trace those who had moved.

For all these reasons, it is not possible to provide a prior specification of the exact manner in which the sample was drawn either from the general population of the city, or from the country as a whole. We have had to rely on post-hoc comparisons. Fortunately, we were able to test the representative nature of the women who returned questionnaires, against the total hospital population. Using the maternity records, we compared the two groups in terms of the most important predictive parameters, including social, obstetric and anaesthetic factors. We also estimated the extent to which the 'non-returning' fraction consisted of women who had moved or, alternatively, women who failed to respond. Fortunately the high response rate (79%) estimated among women still living at the latest known address, or traced through postal re-direction, left little room for substantial response bias in terms of the social and obstetric events of greatest interest.

For these reasons, extrapolations from sample prevalances to population estimates, as essayed in the last section, can be treated with reasonable confidence. The main reason for caution is not so much the sampling difficulties but the dependence of the estimates upon the women's self perceptions, guided by idiosyncratic and socially-related interpretations of the terms used; and upon the varying degrees of motivation which they felt. There was evidence of these problems in the 'background aggregation' phenomenon reported in the previous chapter. However, insofar as we limited our main analytical studies to reports which were adequately dated and appropriately specified, our prevalence estimates should probably be regarded as lower limits.

We have reviewed these technical problems in some detail because similar issues will almost certainly arise in any attempts to repeat this study in other localities. Some of these problems seem inescapable, and perhaps unresolvable, and strict comparisons of prevalences will always be difficult, but we hope to have shown that the approach is capable of producing reasonably robust estimates, and of demonstrating relationships with little ambiguity.

Questionnaire methods

Postal questionnaires are sometimes suspected of producing only 'soft' data. They are also limited in the number and specificity of the questions which can be asked; and by the difficulties of imposing rigorous definitions or overcoming idiosyncratic interpretations. They can be prone to the problems of incomplete response, and of unmeasured and uncontrolled biases between responders and non-responders. However, the latter can be overcome if the response rate is sufficiently high, and the method brings its intrinsic advantages of access to very large amounts of information, speed of operation and relative cheapness. No other method would have been feasible with the number of women required by this form of investigation. Cartwright (1987) has shown and we have confirmed, that post-partum women are well motivated to co-operate, that the response rates are high, and that the respondents exhibit a high accuracy of recall for events associated with their deliveries. This level of accuracy does not necessarily apply however to post-partum symptoms occurring several years previously, which have not already been so precisely 'labelled', and this last point is exacerbated because so few women in fact attended their doctors. This must have contributed to the 'background aggregation' phenomenon, as demonstrated in Chapter 15.

In order to make true comparisons of post-partum symptoms between one part of the country and another, or one hospital and another, exactly the same approaches and questionnaire forms would have to be used. The current questionnaire however was designed against prevalence-expectations far below those actually encountered and several important issues arose only when the results were finally analysed. The form may not therefore by optimal for future comparative purposes. It will be important then to develop and standardise an instrument more closely tailored to the levels of morbidity observed, to the problems now identified, and to the purposes now envisaged.

One major virtue of our investigative design, and one which could not be repeated without having first established the necessary facilities, was the absence of important artefactual correlation between the dependent and the independent variables. This was because the preditor variables had already been recorded using a method totally independent of that used for accessing subsequent health problems. As we have commented in a previous chapter (Chapter 4), population studies which rely upon a single method for recording both the dependent and the independent variables, are more difficult to interpret.

With the benefit of hindsight we would have included two additional sets of questions in the enquiry. The first would be about the circumstances of the previous symptom-occurrences in women who reported that the complaint was not a new one. In particular, any association with previous births is relevant in order to assess the possibility of cumulative injury; also whether the symptoms were associated with the index pregnancy, but had started before delivery. This would have enabled us to be confident that pregnancy-induced symptoms were not referred to and included by some women as post-delivery symptoms (see Chapter 7). Our second area of omission concerned similar symptoms that women had experienced in the past but *not* following this delivery. We enquired about the presence of previous symptoms *only* when the symptom was recorded on this occasion. In future investigations on post-partum morbidity we would recommend that these areas were covered.

Overall, the symptom coverage achieved by this questionnaire, and the response levels, were gratifying; and the quality of reporting was adequate for our purposes. Our results can be taken to confirm again (see Cartwright 1987) the pragmatic validity of this approach as a health survey method.

Associations: predictors: causes?

We pursued our search for the possible causes of health problems through several distinct steps. First, the post-partum prevalences of the different health problems were tabulated against each of the independent variables separately to construct profiles such as those displayed graphically in Figure 10.1, 11.1, 12.1 ... etc. Where two symptoms exhibited substantial overlap, as with urinary frequency and stress incontinence, we first carried out these tabulations for each, irrespective of the presence or absence of the other. We then examine each of them alone: and then the combined symptoms.

The second step was to conduct a form of multivariate analysis – discriminant analysis – in order to determine which of the associations stood up to standardisation against all the others and could be identified as predictors of health problems. The third step consisted of multi-way tabulations designed to seek non-linear or localised relationships which might have escaped the discriminant procedure.

Where all of these methods provided a concordant result, as was the case for the relationship between epidural anaesthesia and subsequent long-term backache, and where there was ancillary evidence to suggest a plausible mechanism, the interpretation was reasonably straightforward and we have postulated a potential causal relationship. In other cases we were more cautious with our interpretations. In general we have suggested ways in which the particular questions could be interrogated by further study.

The statistical reliabilities of all these demonstrated associations were handled by the statistical package in terms of significance tests, notably chi-square and the F-ratio. Each of these can be converted to P-values; expressed as decimal fractions (e.g. 0.01). These values represent the probability that an association could arise purely by chance in a sample, through the random processes involved in drawing it, without there being a real correlation within the population from which the sample was drawn. This is a standard approach.

However, in the context of discriminant (and other multivariate) analysis there is another way in which sampling variation can disturb the reliability of the conclusions based upon a sample. Suppose that two independent variables – for example the duration of the first stage of labour and the duration of the second stage of labour – are themselves highly correlated: and that each of them is separately associated with a particular outcome, such as stress incontinence. Each measure of duration alone would have served as an effective predictor of the symptom, if we had not had a record of the other. In multivariate analysis, where both are examined together, the statistical analytical process will choose the 'best' predictor, and use it to best effect. The 'second-best' predictor may then be redundant. It supplies insufficient *additional* information to be taken into account by the analytical package, and so it is dicarded. The problem, from the point of view of scientific analysis, is that the inevitable random elements in the assembly of the sample may occasionally determine which of the two is chosen as 'best', and which is discarded.

This is a problem mainly related to the examination of fine detail, when the numbers in individual classes becomes smaller. It is for this reason that we have always sought to confirm findings through more than one technical route, combining simple tabulations with several alternative forms of discriminant anslysis, and following up the last results with multi-way cross-tabulations.

These issues are dissected to this extent here because they impinge upon our overall interpretations of the findings – especially the problems of inferring potential simple and multiple determinants of the specific health problems and related groups of problems. This can never be a purely formal, or an objectively verifiable process. It demands the formulation of a broad etiological model, comprising a set of discrete causal hypotheses, linked and in sequence. It also demands access to information other than that on which the statistical analysis was itself based, including neuro-anatomical, nutritional/metabolic and pharmacological knowledge. The essential task is to propose mechanisms which are jointly compatible with the findings as demonstrated, and with this pre-existing knowledge. Preferably the model should provide the *only* way in which the strands of evidence can be reconciled. A satisfactory model will also suggest which of any marginally significant findings can reasonably be accepted, and which of them should be rejected, or subjected to further analysis. We develop these ideas in the next section.

A model etiological framework

In the present instance, where several potential determinants seem to operate, where certain outcomes may depend upon more than one 'cause', and where certain events contribute to more than one outcome, we shall have to construct a global hypothetical framework within which the separate components fit. We must stress that this model is hypothetical, its elements put forward for varying levels of testing.

We begin logically at the beginning, and propose that our hypothetical causal framework for post-partum morbidity be considered as a sequence of three interacting stages. The first set of 'causes' lies in the social and ethnic backgrounds of the women involved: the second in the events, the circumstances and the obstetric and anaesthetic procedures of childbirth: and the third in the post-partum environment. Each set of proposed 'causes' lays the foundation on which the subsequent set of 'causes' then acts; and superimposed upon the whole of this process lie variations in self perceptions of illness, in labelling, and in reporting. We consider the three main stages in turn.

Pre-delivery 'causes'

Several predictors of subsequent morbidity were recorded as present prior to the birth. They include maternal age, parity, social class, marital status and ethnic group. However the characteristics recorded before the birth were generally also present afterwards. It would often be impossible to infer the timing of their action from the statistical correlations alone. Their exact mode of action would anyway sometimes depend on factors which were not observed directly, such as economic and domestic stress, nutritional inadequacies and the physical load of caring for children.

Maternal age was probably relevant to various problems both before, during and after the delivery, but the most direct of the early effects related to stress incontinence. The higher rates of this symptom in older women were present in many different circumstances, including delivery by Caesarean section. As many as one in five primiparae aged 30 or more reported stress incontinence as a new long-term complaint. We postulate that this age component of symptom determination, occurring irrespective of the vaginal passage of the infant, probably operates through a weakened musculature, which might be damaged further during a traumatic delivery, and perhaps recovering less readily than in a younger woman.

Other probable pre-delivery determinants of post-partum morbidity can be related to the previous obstetric history. The only recorded element, in our analysis, was parity; so the relationships are inferred rather than directly measured. Apart from the general artefactual relationships with primparity resulting from selective exclusion of recurring symptoms at higher birth ranks, there was probably an additional form of selection – the so-called 'healthy survivor effect'. This phenomenon has been observed in populations surviving major disasters: and among industrial recruits successfully passing a recruitment selection procedure. Those who are most likely to 'fall ill' are excluded; and those remaining in the sample are those most likely to stay well. In the case of haemorrhoids, the frequency of new occurrences among the so-far-unaffected women decreased at successive birth ranks, suggesting that those who were susceptible to this complication after childbirth, tended to get it after their first delivery. The women who survived the first delivery without it were already selected as a low risk group and this showed when the second baby arrived.

For stress incontinence, however, the 'healthy survivor' effect was not evident. The risk of new symptoms occurring among the unaffected 'survivors' of previous pregnancies, remained fairly constant at successive births. The effect, if it operated here, may have been neutralised, by cumulative injury at successive deliveries. Given the published evidence that neurological injuries play an important part in the genesis of this condition (Snooks et al 1984; 1990 Allen et al 1990) it would not be surprising if successive decrements of neurological functions were to occur at successive deliveries. This is an area demanding further investigation.

We have inferred a nutritionally-related background mechanism, from our findings among the Asian women. This was related to a range of inter-correlated symptoms comprising pain in the arms, pain in the legs, weakness in the arm, weakness in the legs, backache, shoulder-ache and headache. The vitamin B deficiencies commonly observed among Asian women, (Brooke et al 1980; Wharton & Wharton 1989) originating from combinations of dietary idiosyncrasies, dress customs and pigmented skin, make it likely that some of these symptoms are mediated through the occurrence of overt or incipient osteomalacia. This may produce some symptoms before the child is born, or later, after the delivery, as a result of the additional metabolic and physical stresses of the pregnancy, delivery, breast feeding and extra pressures upon the household economy. Nutritional inadequacies might increase susceptibility to the postural stresses of delivery, thus magnifying the risk of backache, with or without the superimposed enhancement effected by an epidural. We may presume that the extra physical loads of later child-care exacerbate the problem yet again.

We paid particular attention, right from the beginning, to the possibility that some women might react excessively to the kinds of questions asked. Some responses might be psychoneurotic or hypochondriacal in type, covering a wide range of different symptoms. We might expect special emphasis upon fatigue, headache and depression. Another style of general response might be focused upon an excessive reaction to pain. It was for these reasons that we included several 'dummy' questions, referring to vaguely defined and relatively trivial symptoms, and others related to several different types of pain. In fact, although there was clear evidence of varying perceptions as to what was a 'reportable' symptom, and although headache and depression and fatigue were associated with the indicators of socio-economic, environmental and physical stress, there was little direct evidence of psychoneurotic reporting. It was limited in scale and did not seem to compromise the validity of our other conclusions. Nor was there direct evidence of differing responses to pain.

Delivery-associated 'causes'

We identified a major group of pelvic symptoms – stress incontinence, urinary frequency and haemorrhoids – which were strongly correlated with indicators of a traumatic vaginal delivery. Caesarean section was generally 'protective'. There were however some differences in detail in the patterns of predictors between stress incontinence, urinary frequency unaccompanied by stress incontinence and haemorrhoids, suggesting that several different mechanisms are involved.

We found evidence in published work (Snook et at 1984; 1986; 1990) that stress incontinence is mediated through neurological injury, presumably ischaemic, a consequence of prolonged 'wedging' of the baby's head, with compression of the pelvic nerves. However we have suggested that the clear maternal age association, even without the vaginal passage of the baby, indicates an additional effect implicating loss of sphincter muscular competence, more pronounced with ageing. Haemorrhoids could scarcely occur through such a mechanism and were more probably due to direct soft tissue injury or localised venous pressure. Urinary frequency in the absence of stress incontinence could plausibly be due to soft tissue injury, but the evidence to support any traumatic delivery-related association at all was weak and its origins might be entirely post-delivery: perhaps infective. This needs examining.

There was some evidence from the different durations and onset times of stress incontinence in older women that an additional effect of increasing age might be to retard recovery. Innervation injuries might also be incremental, worsening with successive deliveries. These factors possibly contributed to the different parity sequences of stress incontinence compared with haemorrhoids. However, this evidence is weak, and for the time being should be regarded only as a pointer towards further investigations.

A second major set of proposed delivery-related symptoms involved the spinal axis. There appeared to be two apparent 'syndromes' here. The first was centred on pain in the back, sometimes extending to the neck, to headache and to tingling in the hands. The second, affecting much smaller numbers of women, was centred on pain in the neck and shoulder, extending to the head and to pain in the arms. The obstetric/anaesthetic associations of the two 'syndromes' differed. The first was related to the use of epidural and spinal anaesthesia, and a long second stage. It was probably mediated through prolonged postural stresses, and the epidural enhancement was effected through loss of muscle tone and the inhibition of discomfort-feedback. The second, less frequent syndrome, was associated with Caesarean section and general anaesthesia, and could be caused by a more acute form of neck injury, the result of positioning for intubation. Both need further investigation.

The hypothesis that backache enhanced by epidural anaesthesia was primarily postural came from several sources. The first was the near-absence of epidural enhancement among women who had an elective Caesarean section; this was limited to women undergoing vaginal deliveries or emergency sections – that is women who underwent a period in labour. The second supporting piece of evidence was adduced from the observation of a similar relationship following the much less frequently used procedure of spinal anaesthesia. Here, the end-site of the injection differs as generally does the duration of the anaesthesia. Spinal anaestheisa is a single-shot procedure not entailing the passage of an indwelling catheter. Despite the differences, the patterns of association were the same. The third piece of evidence was the high rate, one in ten, of backache occurring after deliveries without an epidural; epidurals could not be the unique determinant. The independent relationship between backache and longer second stage of labours, without epidurals, was consistent with this hypothesis.

Among Caucasians the backache extended to neckache and headache together with tingling in the arms. The neckache is almost certainly a secondary symptom, following on from the postural mitigation of the backache, while tingling in the hands and fingers could be a neurological consequence of the secondary cervical problem. In Asians – in whom the prevalence of the general 'spinal-axis syndrome' was doubled – it was accompanied also by a fourfold excess of pain and weakness in the arms and pain and weakness in the legs. The pain and weakness might be osteomalacia symptoms, with pre-delivery origins, and this would account for the extreme clustering in Asians. The risk of postural backache could be enhanced in women with osteomalacia, although not uniquely dependent upon it.

Postnatal depression/anxiety showed several delivery-related associations but they were not clearly consistent with those of the major pelvic symptoms or with a hypothesis of vaginal trauma. There was a relationship with the duration of labour, but mainly for first stage: and Caesarean sections and smaller babies were associated with higher, rather than lower, symptom rates. Insofar as the determinants of depression could be inferred from this data set, it reflected a combination of early maternal age and post-partum social pressures.

There were also two clear delivery-related predictors of extreme tiredness which we had not anticipated but for which there was a possible explanation, one much more tentative than the other. The first was an association between post-partum haemorrhage and extreme tiredness. The fatigue here often started in the first post-delivery week, and generally resolved within a year, and we therefore suppose it to be a symptom of consequent undetected or inadequately treated anaemia. Some women had haemoglobin estimations below 10gms per 100ml recorded in their case-notes as a complicating factor of the puerperium but we do not know what proportion of the remainder were measured or not. However the critical factor was a record of a post-partum haemorrhage rather than a record of anaemia.

The other delivery-related association of fatigue, was the use of inhalation analgesia – nitrous oxide – for pain relief during labour. The associations were similar to those for post-partum haemorrhage and we first enquired whether nitrous oxide might cause anaemia through binding to haemoglobin, causing methaemoglobinaemia and subsequent loss of red blood cells. However, there seems to be no evidence of this. One possible explanation is through another known pharmacological mechanism in which nitrous oxide interferes with the utilisation of Vitamin B12. (Baden et al 1984; Koblin and Tomersen 1990) Unlike post-partum haemorrhage the fatigue associated with nitrous oxide usage was *not* of immediate onset and tended to develop in the period two to four weeks after the birth, a timing which could be compatible with this mechanism. However interpretation is very tentative, since the evidence relating to nitrous oxide and Vitamin B12 is chiefly animal-based. The matter requires further study.

Finally we noted two perplexing delivery related associations among the osteomalacia-like musculo-skeletal symptoms. There were significant relationships (although small numerically) between tranquillisers given during labour and pain in the legs; and between the use of pethidine and neckache, weakness in the legs and tingling in the hands. Again, there may be a possible pharmacological explanation. Many tranquillisers – along with barbiturates and anticonvulsants – stimulate intra-cellular production of microsomal oxidases. These enzymes dispose of the drugs which stimulate their production, reducing the efficiency of the drugs and demanding larger doses. However, the oxidases stimulated by one drug also degrade others: and Vitamin D is included among them. Osteomalacia is a long-recognised complication of anticonvulsant therapy. It might be possible, although this is extremely tentative and would need direct study, that tranquillisers given even for a short time could convert a marginal osteomalacia to an overt one, through this route. There was no evidence that pethidine stimulates oxidases, but it appears upon enquiry that pethidine administration was usually accompanied by unrecorded anti-emetic preparations of the phenothiazine group which could also have the same effect.

Post-partum environmental 'causes'

Most of the social and domestic circumstances identifiable as pre-delivery hazards were still present after the birth, and for many it was probably the additional stress of caring for the child afterwards that precipitated the symptoms. Most of these circumstances and their postulated effects have been inferred indirectly rather than observed.

Our study of frequent headaches and migraine showed that where these symptoms occurred alone, unaccompanied by backache, they were related especially to inferred stresses within the post-partum environment. These headaches were more common among women under 25 years who had given birth to a second or subsequent baby. Their onsets were not necessarily immediate, and sometimes began more than three months after the delivery. Lower social class was an additional independent predictor and there was a (crude) association with unemployment of the husband. A reasonable hypothesis would be that this form of headache reflects the additional burdens upon young mothers of coping and caring for two or more children under domestic, environmental and economic stress.

Postnatal depression without a concomitant report of fatigue followed a similar age pattern; it was also more frequent among women under 25, although this time in both parity groups. Asian women had lower symptom rates, both for depression without fatigue and for headache unaccompanied by backache. This is compatible with the extended family networks and community-based social support systems typical of this ethnic group, such that the post-delivery stresses of child-care are felt less severely.

Extreme post-partum fatigue mainly occurring without depression was a feature of older mothers, worst of all in those who had delivered their first baby at 30 years or more. This age association, especially the first birth effect, might be explained partly as a labelling bias, the older new mothers finding the whole experience more of a shock. However, it is also likely that older mothers do indeed have less stamina, and truly experience greater fatigue.

The unmarried state, another potential source of post-partum stress, was a major predictor of depression and fatigue; especially occurring together, and of the longest lasting symptoms, those still unresolved at the time of our enquiry. Our record of marital status was taken at antenatal booking, and some women would have married by the time of the birth, while others would be living with the baby's father, as if married. Among those who lived alone after the delivery, the rates of depression and fatigue were probably greater still.

There were two further indicators of a potentially stressful postnatal environment associated with depression and fatigue: twins, and breast feeding.

It is scarcely surprising that the mothers of twins should report greater levels of fatigue but the association with postnatal depression was less obvious, and does not seem to have been previously documented. Our breast feeding data were unsatisfactory, referring only to the patterns at the time of hospital discharge, but here too there are plausible mechanisms, through the constant ties and lack of sleep arising from the inability to share feeding responsibility, especially night feeds. Like the unmarried association these complaints were often of long duration.

In contrast with headache or depression or fatigue, the major pelvic symptoms (incontinence, frequency, haemorrhoids) showed no specific associations with any elements of the post-partum environment on which we had information. Except for maternal age, all the predictors of these symptoms, were related specifically to the delivery. We should not however abandon the notion that post delivery factors, such as medical intervention and life-style advice, could affect their resolution. Pelvic floor exercises might improve or cure stress incontinence: or dietary habits might influence the resolution of haemorrhoids or limit the risk at the next pregnancy. However these again must all be the subjects of further investigations.

Backache, and the wider epidural-related spinal-axis syndrome, also exhibited their closest associations with elements of the delivery itself although they were different in detail. Unlike the pelvic symptoms, however the occurrence and persistence of these spinal-axis symptoms showed the likely additional existence of a relationship with the postnatal environment. Backache following an epidural did not necessarily start until several weeks after the delivery. This suggests that for some women the epidural-related postural stresses of delivery only resulted in back pain together with an additional post-partum trigger. We have no specific information on what these could be, although there are many obvious possible hazards in the care of a young baby. They include carrying the baby about; bending and lifting carrycots, car seats and heavy loads of washing; and sitting in potentially damaging positions for feeding, especially breast feeding. These same factors probably also apply to the triggering of back pain among women after a delivery without an epidural.

There was one notable exception to this pattern of delayed symptomatology. Where backache and headache occurred together after an epidural, the symptoms almost always started immediately, pre-empting any opportunities for the post-partum environment to impinge.

Conclusions

This chapter has served several purposes. One was to review the main findings of earlier chapters and to relate them to each other. Another, was to extrapolate the results to the population at large and to estimate the consequent burdens upon the women of this country, and upon the health-care services. A third was to review and discuss technical matters encountered during the research, and of interest to other researchers seeking to undertake similar studies to confirm or to question the main results. The last was to formulate a hypothetical etiological framework capable of explaining and accommodating the different findings within a global model: in particular a model capable of indicating needs for additional enquiries and of pointing the way towards subsequent interventions.

Chapter 17 – Implications for Action

The results of our investigation, both the basic findings and their wider interpretations, implicate action at several different levels. Some of our conclusions are more well-founded and suggest obvious solutions, while others demand more cautious progress towards preventive or therapeutic programmes through randomised trials conducted on an evaluative basis. In other cases the guiding hypotheses are more tentative still, and the inferences require confirmation through additional data sets collected for specific purposes.

Before that, the general range of findings needs to be confirmed; again at several different levels. First, prevalence surveys should be carried out in different parts of the country using a variety of sampling-frames, and linking the results with pre-existing social, obstetric and anaesthetic data both in the manner exemplified here and using alternative methodologies. Second, the specific post-partum findings need to be confirmed at more detailed levels using specialised questionnaires randomised methods, direct interview and sometimes medical examination – for example in relation to back injury or serum chemistry. Third, we need more information on the severity of the recorded symptoms and their impacts upon the lives of the women and their families. Finally, we need much more information on the sequential patterns of the development and resolution of different symptoms across successive pregnancies.

At the level of medical practice it seems also clear that the traditional six-week postnatal examination can no longer be regarded as a satisfactory termination for this episode of care. Its traditional format requires supplementation along the lines indicated by the data on the onsets and durations of the different symptoms. For many women, perhaps all, a further enquiry covering a schedule of specific points is indicated not just at six weeks but at some later date, for example at six months. There is probably additional scope for specific antenatal enquiry on the conditions which lay the ground for the development of such problems as nutritional deficiency or depression and fatigue.

There are also many specific actions or proposed actions to be prescribed in relation to particular symptoms and 'syndromes': and we discuss them under separate headings, below.

Backache, headache and musculo-skeletal symptoms

The potential determinants of these symptoms were dominated by epidural anaesthesia and Asian ethnic group. There was a separate but much smaller grouping with particular emphasis upon pain in the neck and shoulders which seemed to be associated with Caesarean section and general anaesthesia.

Detailed analysis of the data permitted the nomination of three other inferred determinants, namely nutritional deficiencies, postural stresses during labour, and lifting stresses in the three months following delivery. Each of these invites further research and each suggests potential remedies.

The priorities allocated to these actions will depend to a large extent upon the severity of these particular complaints, a point on which we currently have no information. We know that many were of long duration, and often chronic, but their effects upon the quality of life is not known. Better information is needed, especially where we have shown that symptoms seem to be related to particular procedures. It will influence the priorities to be placed upon the research and upon the design of policies for intervention, as well as informing the choice which a woman makes. If, for example, backaches after epidural were shown to be continuous and extremely painful, as well as frequent, the numbers opting for this procedure would presumably diminish; whereas slight and intermittent pain would affect the choice much less.

A second major research requirement springs from the observation of the striking prevalence of post-partum musculo-skeletal problems among Asian women. Backache, headache and limb symptoms, particularly pains and weakness, were increased, independently of epidural anaesthesia, but increased yet more when this had been undertaken. We have proposed that this probably follows upon vitamin-D deficiency and resulting osteomalacia. A first requirement is that the hypothesis be tested directly. If this is confirmed, then dietary supplements sometime during the pregnancy might be sufficient, (Brooke et al 1980; Cockburn et al 1980; Mallet et al 1986) although an earlier detection and amelioration of the problem might prove necessary. Preventive regimes such as these require careful and detailed monitoring and should preferably be conducted within the framework of a randomised controlled experiment. Although this problem was greatest among Asians, there might be similar mechanisms among some Caucasian women; and this too requires further research.

The third set of opportunities for research and action concerning backache and its associated symptoms relates to intra-partum processes. The two main points of potential enquiry and intervention concern posture during labour, and the detailed management-regimes used for epidural anaesthesia, general anaesthesia and spinal anaesthesia.

The postural component demands detailed observation of the postures actually adopted and imposed, and a range of experimental interventions involving modified postures, the imposition of time limits in particular positions, and prescribed and assisted movement. Effective interventions may include the use of specially designed supports, with separate approaches required for vaginal and Caesarean deliveries, and for epidural and general anaesthesias.

Epidural anaesthesia for pain relief in labour, during the study period, typically consisted of administering a standard volume of local anaesthetic of varying concentrations, sufficient to produce sensory block but also inducing a degree of motor block. This is repeated as required. There has been a trend more recently to aim for barely sufficient analgesia for labour, thus leaving the woman with some capacity for movement. However, the response to a given dose varies in different women and it is not always possible to achieve continued mobility. But there is clear scope for further experimentation, and for developing techniques which employ the minimum necessary levels of anaesthesia, compatible with acceptable pain relief perhaps combined with systemic analgesics; and perhaps for limiting the duration of anaesthesia insofar as this is possible. Retrospective investigations on the relationships between the levels and durations of anaesthesia in this sample, and the risk of subsequent backache, are already underway. Non-coded anaesthetic records for the women included in this sample are still available and will be linked with the present data set.

Prolonged labour, the last of the important intra-partum predictors of backache, presents a less tractable problem. However, the duration of the first stage predicts the duration of the second stage, and the duration of each predicts the risk of backache. These relationships can perhaps serve as practical risk-markers, which can direct special attention towards prevention through other means.

The remaining questions of concern in this group of symptoms relate to the post-partum period. There are two main questions. Can later-onset backache be prevented in the interval immediately after delivery? and once backache has started can it be more effectively treated? Both of these questions, together with the intra-partum postural problems, might be amenable to post-hoc physiotherapy. Even without an epidural, one in ten women experienced newly occurring long-term backache. Investigations directed towards the prevention and treatment of backache in the higher risk groups might well lead to effective action, with respect to back pain, for the lower risk non-epidural deliveries.

These questions will best be answered, ultimately, through the use of randomised controlled intervention trials, for both preventive and therapeutic regimes, and incorporating physiotherapy, modifications of delivery and anaesthetic procedures, education of women and their partners on the avoidance of higher risk activities, and perhaps drug therapies as well. The immediate requirement is for intermediate studies based upon more detailed observations of the origins of these symptoms, so that useful interventions can more effectively be formulated, and trials more effectively designed.

Finally, long-term headache occurred in two additional circumstances. First, and implicating post-partum environmental stresses, headache in the absence of backache was associated with early maternal age, multiparity and lower social class, and as such is beyond the scope of action on the part of the health services. Second, it appeared as an extremely low frequency problem after either spinal anaesthesia or accidental dural tap. Only nine women were affected but this represented 26% of the 34 recorded spinal headaches, and it was also noted in the study by Kitzinger (see Chapter 8) as a long-term effect of epidurals. Confirmation of this finding is required.

Bladder symptoms

The main proposed determinants of stress incontinence alone, and of stress incontinence accompanied by urinary frequency, were almost all intra-partum. There was also a powerful association with increasing maternal age, both after vaginal and Caesarean section deliveries. It has been suggested that stress incontinence with or without frequency was sometimes determined by an ischaemic innervation injury (Snooks et al 1984; 1986; 1990) but we think that this cannot provide the full explanation. There may be an additional contributory effect of direct injury to the perineal and sphincter muscles. The age relationship, following Caesarean section, with its reduced but still finite risk tends to confirm its independence from nerve injuries of this type. This demands detailed study.

If this hypothesis of a complex of alternative and additive pathways is confirmed then it is difficult to see possible interventions directed at the determinants of these symptoms either singly, or en bloc. Advancing age cannot be altered; bigger babies are for other reasons an advantage; and although a long second stage labour might be shortened by forceps, this too seems to carry a risk in some cases. Caesarean section, which offers considerable protection against stress incontinence, would scarcely be justified on these grounds alone, and it too carries additional hazards. If there are any potentially effective interventions, then they will probably have to be directed mainly towards mechanisms other than those accessed by our enquiry.

There might be scope for intra-partum intervention in relation to the quality of the repair of the perineum. Most (81%) women with vaginal deliveries in our sample had either lacerations or an episiotomy. Very few escaped one or the other unless they had a section. The case-notes contained only crude and uncoded assessments of the severity of the perineal injury and contained no details regarding the experience of the person carrying out the repair, or any information of the quality of the repair. This is an area which merits attention, although it is the measure of prevalence, rather than the detection of associations with recorded procedures, which says so.

The most obvious initial area for investigation and action relates to instruction on pelvic floor exercises designed to strengthen perineal muscles. In many maternity units women are routinely seen by physiotherapy staff and given leaflets and/or invited to attend a class; but for the first-time mother, the first few days after birth are a time when many new skills have to be learned and those relating to the care of the baby seem of more immediate concern. After later births, women are often discharged from hospital so quickly that they may not even get a reminder about the necessity for these exercises. Beyond these operational issues lies another major question – the question whether perineal floor exercises are indeed efficacious in preventing or alleviating long-term stress-incontinence (Sleep and Grant 1987).

The best assistance towards these health education processes which our study might supply, lies in the identification of high risk categories of women, enabling a concentration of effort towards their particular benefit. Women who are informed that due to their age, length of delivery and size of baby, they are at much greater risk than aveage of suffering subsequent stress incontinence and perhaps urinary frequency, are likely to take more note of advice given about remedial exercises. The individual motivation might be even greater if women are made aware that the problem, once established, is frequently permanent. Many women know about the problem of leakage of urine in certain circumstances after childbirth, but do not know that this so often becomes chronic.

Urinary frequency without stress incontinence affected 2% of the sample. It was largely unrelated to intra-partum predictors, and there were no social predictors either. The data suggest that we should be looking for an entirely different mechanism, possible post-partum. The introduction of low grade bacterial infections to the bladder must seem a likely candidate, with ample opportunity for this to occur around delivery. For some women the post-partum problem may be an outcome of infection present during pregnancy. These hypotheses need to be investigated: especially since there is an obvious and straightforward solution, in the form of routine urine-culture, and administration of antibiotics.

Haemorrhoids

This problem resembled stress incontinence with or without urinary frequency to the extent that the proposed determinants were mainly related to the delivery itself. In points of detail however, the picture differed and the findings would suggest soft tissue injuries rather than neurological injuries: a hypothesis reinforced by the difficulty in suggesting a neurological mechanism. Haemorrhoids can start first during pregnancy and the symptoms can occur before delivery. Some of those noted after the birth might have in fact started earlier and been aggravated to the extent of becoming symptomatic, rather than initiated, by delivery trauma. Be this as it may, the situation resembles that for incontinence in that it is difficult to suggest potentially effective interventions directed towards the precipitating intra-partum determinants. Again, we have to consider factors outside the direct range of our enquiry.

One such area relates to diet; and the much lower rates of this symptom among Asian women provides some indirect evidence that dietary differences affect susceptibilities. The picture of reducing risks after successive births also implies that where women are susceptible to haemorrhoids, they will tend to occur after the first baby. Women who have not developed haemorrhoids after the first baby are those who are least susceptible. As with the bladder symptoms, these possibilities and necessities arise from our observations regarding the previously undocumented high prevalence of this condition together with its tendency to become chronic, rather than any demonstrations of direct associations with the traumas of delivery. At this stage, our recommendations must be for additional special enquiries, rather than immediate action.

The other necessary area for research – for all of these pelvic symptoms – relates to their severity. We now know something of their frequency, their potential determinants and their tendency towards chronicity, but like the musculo-skeletal symptoms we know little of their severity and the extent to which they impinge on the women's overall health and well-being.

Depression and extreme fatigue

Depression and fatigue exhibited multiple associations which appeared sometimes to act in an additive manner. It was difficult to localise particular mechanisms of these symptoms or to award them priorities. It was equally difficult in many cases to think of ways of influencing them: such factors as maternal age, unmarried status, and twins are in most cases beyond the scope of health-service intervention.

The detailed psychopathology of postnatal depression is clearly complex and a full dissection of the etiology of the condition is clearly beyond the powers of the data assembled here. However, the combination of depression with extreme fatigue was strongly associated with unmarried status, with twins (both especially for prolonged symptoms) and with breast feeding; sufficient to suggest that at least in some cases, the problem arises through relentless physical exhaustion and that it is this which sometimes leads to subsequent depression. With sufficiently careful routine assessment it might be possible to identify women living in circumstances likely to promote this sequence of events, and to channel necessary assistance. In some cases it might be justified even to discourage breast feeding.

Previous studies (Adler, Cox 1983; Dalton 1971) have shown breast feeding to be a predictor of postnatal depression, focusing upon the hypothesis of a hormonal mechanism. The present investigation also points towards a hypothesis based upon an additional 'burden-of-care', mediated through the constant and inescapable ties imposed by breast feeding through fatigue, and through an inability to share responsibility especially for night feeding. Women who were unmarried and who breast-fed their infants reported higher rates of extreme tiredness than when either factor was present singly.

Straightforward fatigue, without accompanying depression, was predicted both by post-partum haemorrhage and by inhalation analgesia. For the first of these there seems to be an obvious explanation: and an obvious solution. The early discharge of women after delivery might mean that some women do not have their haemoglobin measured at all, or after a time-interval sufficient for post-haemorrhage haemodilution to have taken place. Those who are tested and found to have anaemia are generally provided with only an initial supply of ferrous sulphate tablets and the general practitioner is expected to replenish them where necessary. There are therefore several points at which the system can break down. For whatever reasons, our data suggest that there is a significant degree of undiagnosed and/or untreated post-partum anaemia, which could so easily be remedied.

It would be surprising if this problem was limited exclusively to women who had a record of a PPH. It might be prudent for all women to receive a routine haemoglobin test at an appropriate time. This aspect of the post-natal service should be monitored, and women with anaemia should be followed up.

The relationship between fatigue and nitrous-oxide inhalation analgesia was a surprising one and one that needs detailed consideration. There is pharmacological evidence that nitrous oxide interferes with Vitamin B_{12} metabolism, and the fatigue associated with nitrous oxide certainly exhibited a delayed onset and eventual resolution, as we might then expect. However, the toxicological evidence in relation to pregnancy is based upon rats rather than humans and the question whether the typical intermittent exposure to inhalation analgesia in labour could feasibly produce such a delayed and prolonged effect in women, needs to be answered.

Less frequent effects of childbirth

Our investigation revealed a number of other less frequent problems demanding further enquiry. The first related to hypertension. There was evidence from the women's replies that hypertension of pregnancy did not always resolve as quickly as is generally believed. However, there is much scope for misunderstanding, such that it would be unwise to speculate on the existence of the phenomenon, let alone look for causes, without carrying out further investigations. We should first review the detailed coding of a diagnosis of hypertension in the maternity records taking note of the recorded pressures. We should also conduct investigations in which post-partum blood pressure is actually measured, rather than relying on women's own reports.

Second, a number of generalised 'neurological' symptoms – dizziness, visual disturbances and buzzing in the ears – were associated with various forms of anaesthesia and analgesia. They were very infrequent and possible reporting bias could provide an explanation, but this might repay further investigation.

Finally, there was a small group of women reporting localised paraesthaesias, or loss of sensation in various different parts of the body, related to particular procedures, notably epidural anaesthesia, forceps and Caesarean section. The question of localised neurological injuries arising from these procedures, although affecting extremely small numbers and probably not excessively troublesome, also deserves more detailed enquiry.

Last words

Finally, and whatever the outcomes of these proposed endeavours might be, it would seem essential from now onwards to devise new recording schedules, and to collect systematic information on the types of longer term post-partum problems described in this study. This requires the same care and uniformity as that commonly undertaken in relation to immediate maternity care. It should make provision for a planned system of selective postnatal discharge, which for many women would require additional reviews at six months, and for some women beyond that time.

References

Adler E. M. and Cox J. L. (1983). 'Breast feeding and postnatal depression.' *J. of Psychomatic Res.* **27**, 2, 139-144.

Allen R. E., Hasker G. L., Smith A.R.B., Warrell D. W. (1990) Pelvic floor damage and childbirth: a neurophysiological study, Brit J of *Obstet & Gynaec* **97**, 770-79

Baden J.M., Serra M. and Mazze R. I. (1984). 'Inhibition of fetal methionine synthase by nitrous oxide.' *Brit. J. Anaesth.* **56**, 523-526.

Berg G., Hammar M., Muller-Nielsen J., Linden U. and Thorblad J. (1988). 'Low back pain during pregnancy.' *Obstet. & Gynae.* **71**, 1, 71-75.

Bergqvist A, Bergqvist D, Lindhagen A. and Mätzsch T. (1990) Late symptoms after pregnancy-related deep vein thrombosis, Brit J of *Obstet. & Gynae.* **97**, 338-41.

Brandon S. (1983). 'Depression after childbirth.' *Health Visitor* **56**, 13-15.

Brockinton I. and Cox-Roper A. (1988). 'The nosology of puerperal mental illness.' Chap. 1. in Kumar R. and Brockington I. (Eds.) *Motherhood and Mental Illness.* Butterworth and Co., Cambridge.

Brooke O. G., Brown I.R.F., Bone C.D.M., Carter N.D., Cleeve H.J.W., Maxwell J. D., Robinson V. P. and Winder S. M. (1980) Vitamin D supplements in pregnant Asian women: effects on calcium status and fetal growth, *BMJ*, 15 Mar, 751-754.

Brownridge P. (1983). 'The management of headache following accidental dural puncture in obstetric patients.' *Anaesth. Intens. Care.* **11**, 4-15.

Cartwright A. (1987). 'Monitoring maternity services by postal questionnaire to mothers.' *Health Trends* **19**, 19-20.

Clayton S. G., Lewis T.L.T, Pinker G. D (Eds.) (1985). *Obstetrics by Ten Teachers*, 14th Ed, Edward Arnold.

Cockburn F, Belton N. R., Purvis R. J., Giles M. M., Brown J. K, Turner T. L., Wilkinson E. M., Forfar J.O., Barrie W. J. M., McKay G. S., Pocock S. J., (1980) Maternal Vitamin D intake and mineral metabolism in mothers and their newborn infants, *BMJ*, 5 July. 11-14

Cox J. L., Connor Y. M. and Kendall R. E. (1982). 'Prospective study of the psychiatric disorders of childbirth.' *Brit. J. of Psych.* **140,** 111-117.

Crawford J. S. (1972). 'Lumbar epidural block in labour: a clinical analysis.' *Brit. J. Anaesth.* **44,** 66-74.

Crawford J.S. (1985a). *Principles and practice of obstetric anaesthesia.* 5th Ed. Oxford. Blackwell Scientific.

Crawford J. S. (1985b). 'Some maternal complications of epidural analgesia for labour.' *Anaesthesia* **40,** 1219-25.

Dalton K. (1971). 'Prospective study into puerperal depression.' *Brit. J. Psych.* **118,** 689-92.

Feggetter P. and Gath D. (1981). 'Non-psychotic psychiatric disorders in women one year after childbirth.' *J. of Psychosomatic Res.* **25,** 369-72.

Gelder M. (1978). 'Hormones and post-partum depression.' In Salder M. (Ed.) *Mental illness in pregnancy and the puerperium.* Oxford, Oxford University Press.

Gordon R. E., Kapostins E. E. and Gordon K. K. (1965). 'Factors in post-partum emotional adjustment.' *Obstetrics and Gynaecology* **25,** 158-66.

Grove L. H. (1973). 'Backache, headache and bladder dysfunction after delivery.' *Brit. J. Anaesth.* **45,** 1147-49.

Hall M. H. (1991). The Health of the Nation: responses. Health of pregnant women, *BMJ* **303,** 460-462.

Hemmink: E. (1986) Effect of Caesarean Section on fertility and abortions. *J. Reprod. Med.* **86,** 620-24.

Hibbard B. M. (1988). Principles of Obstetrics, London, Butterworths.

Hibbard B. M. and Scott D. B. (1990). 'The availability of epidural anaesthesia and analgesia in obstetrics.' *Brit. J. of Obstet. & Gynae.* **97,** 402-405.

Iffy L. Y. and Kaminetzky H. A. (Eds.) (1981). Principles and Practice of Obstetrics and Perinatology, Vol 2, New York, J Wiley and Sons.

Jacobon L., Kaij L. and Nilsson A. (165). 'Post-partum mental disorders in an unselected sample; frequency of symptoms and disposing factors.' *BMJ* **1,** 1640-43.

Jacoby A. (1987). 'Women's preferences for and satisfaction with current procedures in childbirth – findings from a national study.' *Midwifery* **3**, 117-24.

Jolleys J. (1988). 'Reported prevalence of urinary incontinence in women in a general practice.' *BMJ* **296,** 7 May, 1330-1302.

Katz J. and Adinis S. J. (1980). 'Current Concepts Review: Complications of spinal and epidural anaesthesia.' *J. of Bone & Joint Surgery* **62A,** No. 7., 1219-1222.

Kendall R. E. Rennie D., Clark J. A. and Dean C. (1981). 'The social and obstetric correlates of psychiatric admission in the puerperium.' *Psychol. Med.* **11,** 351-59.

Kitzinger S. (1987). *Some women's experiences of epidurals. A descriptive study.* National Childbirth Trust. London.

Knor E. R. (Ed.) (1987). Decision Making in Obstetrical Nursing, Toronto, Decker Inc.

Koblin D. D. and Tomerson B. W. (1990). 'Dimethylthiourea, A Hydroxyl Radical Scavenger, impedes the inactivation of methionine synthase by nitrous oxide in mice.' *Brit. J. of Anaesth.* **64,** 214-223.

Kumar R. and Robson K. M. (1984). 'A prospective study of emotional disorders in childbearing women.' *Brit. J. of Psych.* **144,** 35-47.

Llewellyn-Jones D. (1990). Fundamentals of Obstetrics and Gynaecology. Vol 1. 5th Ed, London, Faber and Faber.

MacArthur C. and Wakefield J. (1978). 'Mixed sex wards'. *Health and Social Service Journal,* **4593,** May 26, A21-24.

MacArthur C., Newton J. R. and Knox E. G. (1985). 'Effects of anti-smoking health education on infant size at birth: a randomised controlled trial.' *Brit. J. Obstet. & Gynae.* **94,** 295-300.

MacArthur C., Lewis M., Knox E. G. and Crawford J. S. (1990). 'Epidural anaesthesia and long-term backache after childbirth.' *BMJ* **301,** 9-12.

Mallet E., Gugi B., Brunelle P., Henocq A., Basuyau J. P., Lemeur H., (1986) Vitamin D supplementation in pregnancy: A randomised trial of two methods, *Obstet & Gynaecol,* **68,** 300-304.

Martin C. (1987). 'Monitoring maternity services by postal questionnaire: congruity between mothers' reports and their obstetric records.' *Statistics in Med.* **6,** 613-627.

Martin M. E. (1977). 'A maternity hospital study of psychiatric illness associated with childbirth.' *Irish J. of Med. Sci,* **146,** 239-44.

Oakley A. (1980). *Women confined: towards a sociology of childbirth.* Oxford. Martin Robertson.

O'Hara M. W. and Zekoski E. M. (1988). *Post-partum depression: a comprehensive review.* Chap. 2. in Kumar R. and Brockington I. (Eds.) op cit.

OPCS (1986). *Hospital In-patient Enquiry. Maternity Tables 1977-1981.* HMSO.

OPCS (1988). *Hospital In-patient Enquiry. Maternity Tables 1982-1985.* HMSO.

OPCS (1989). *Birth Statistics. Review of the Registrar General on births and patterns of family building in England and Wales 1987* HMSO.

Paykel E. S., Emms E. M., Fletcher J. and Rassaby E. S. (1980). 'Life events and social support in puerperal depression.' *Brit. J. Psych.* **136,** 339-46.

Pitt B. (1968). 'Atypical depression following childbirth.' *Brit. J. Psych.* **114,** 1325-1335.

Pitt B. (1973). 'Maternity blues.' *Brit. J. Psych.* **122,** 431-33.

Playfair H. R. and Gowers J. I. (1981). 'Depression following childbirth – a search for predictive signs.' *J. of Roy. Coll. of Gen. Pract.* **31,** 201-208.

Ramanathan S. (1988). *Obstetric anaesthesia.* Lea and Febiger, Philadelphia.

Sleep J., Grant A., Garcia J., Elbourne D., Spencer J. and Chalmers I. (1984). 'West Berkshire perineal management trial.' *BMJ* **289,** 587-90.

Sleep J. and Grant A. (1987). 'West Berkshire perineal management trial: three year follow-up.' *BMJ* **295,** 749-751.

Sleep J. and Grant A. (1987). 'Pelvic floor exercises in postnatal care.' *Midwifery* **3,** 158-64.

Snooks S. J., Swash M., Setchell M. and Henry M. M. (1984). 'Injury to innervation of pelvic floor sphincter musculature in childbirth.' *Lancet*, Sept. **8**, 546-550.

Snooks, S. J., Swash M., Henry M. M. and Setchell M. (1986). 'Risk factors in childbirth causing damage to the pelvic floor innervation.' *Int. J. Colorect. Dis.* **1**, 20-24.

Snooks S. J., Swash M., Mathers S. G. and Henry M. M. (1990). 'Effect of vaginal delivery on the pelvic floor: a 5-year follow-up.' *Brit. J. Surg.* **77**, 1358-60.

Stein G. S. (1981). 'Headaches in the first postpartum week and their relationship to migraine.' *Headache* **21**, 201-205.

Stein G. S., Morton J., Marsh A., Collins W., Branch C., Desaga U. and Ebeling J. (1984). 'Headaches after childbirth.' *Acta. Neurol. Scand.* **69**, 74-79.

Sturman S. and Beevers D. G. (1990) General medical problems of UK Asians, Ch 9. In McAvoy B.R., and Donaldson L. J., Health Care for Asians, Oxford Medical Publ. Oxford Univ. Press.

Thomas T. M., Plymat K. R., Blannin J. and Meade T. W. (1980). 'Prevalence of urinary incontinence.' *BMJ* **281**, 1243-45.

Tod E. D. M. (1964). 'Puerperal depression.' *Lancet* **2**, 1264-66.

Wang L. P., Fog J., and Bove M. (1987) Transient hearing loss following spinal anaesthesia, *Anaesthesia*, **42**, 1258-63.

Watson J. P., Elliott S. A., Rugg A. J. and Brough D. I. (1984). 'Psychiatric disorder in pregnancy and the first postnatal year.' *Brit. J. Psych.* **144**, 453-62.

Wharton P. and Wharton B. (1989) Nutrition of Asian children: fetus and newborn. Ch 29. In Cruickshank J. K. and Beeven D. G., Ethnic Factors in Health and Disease, Wright, London.

Yarnell J. W. G., Voyle G. J., Richards C. J. and Stephenson T. P. (1981). 'The prevalence and severity of urinary incontinence in women.' *J. Epid. & Comm. Hlth.* **35**, 71-74.

Yarnell J. W. G., Voyle G. J., Sweetnam P. M., Milbank J., Richards C. J. and Stephenson T. P. (1982). 'Factors associated with urinary incontinence in women.' *J. Epid. & Comm. Hlth.* **36**, 58-63.

SURVEY OF MOTHERS' HEALTH

1. Could you please tell us how many babies you have had, when you had them, which hospital you had them in and whether you had a Caesarean section?

	Birthdate	Name of hospital	Did you have a Caesarean section? (YES/NO)
1st baby			
2nd baby			
3rd baby			
4th baby			
Others			

2. When you had the babies, what did you have to help the pain? Please tick everything you had.

	Nothing	Gas/Air	Pethidine Injection	Epidural	Relaxation Exercises
1st baby					
2nd baby					
3rd baby					
4th baby					
Others					

THE FOLLOWING QUESTIONS ARE ABOUT THE BABY YOU HAD ON

3. What did you think about the pain relief you had when you had your baby born on the above date? If you had any of the following, please tick what you thought.

	I was fully satisfied	It only helped	It was no good	It deprived me of pleasure of giving birth	Other (please say what)
Gas/Air					
Pethidine Injection					
Epidural					
Relaxation					

4. Have you had any major illnesses or operations since you had your baby born on the date above?

YES ☐   NO ☐

If YES, could you tell us what you had and when you had it?

P.T.O. →

263

5. We would like to know if you have had any of the following conditions since having your baby born on the date mentioned earlier. For each condition please tell us if you have had it or not by placing a tick in the column headed 'YES' or 'NO'. Every time you have ticked 'YES', please go on to answer questions a, b, c, d and e.

Condition	NO	YES	a. Did you have this condition before the baby's birth? (YES/NO)	b. How long after having the baby did it start or come back?	c. After how long did you stop having it?	d. Did you go to the doctor? (YES/NO)	e. What treatment did you have?
Frequent headaches							
Neck ache							
Shoulder ache							
Ache in the middle of back							
Ache at the bottom of back							
Pain in arms							
Pain in legs							
Weakness in arms							
Weakness in legs							
Bowel upsets							
Tingling in hands or fingers							
Tingling in feet or toes							
Buzzing in ears							
Flashing lights/spots before eyes							
Dizziness/fainting							
Migraine							
Indigestion							
Pass urine very often							
Hard to hold urine when jump, sneeze, etc.							
High blood pressure							
Piles							
Varicose veins							
Dental problems							
Depression/anxiety							
Extreme tiredness							
Other (please say what)							

The Birmingham Maternity Hospital

Queen Elizabeth Medical Centre Edgbaston Birmingham B15 2TG.
021-472 1377 Ext:

Dear Madam,

We have a record that you had a baby in our hospital on

We are carrying out a survey of any later health problems which might occur
in women who have had babies.   We are also interested in the different
types of pain relief (if any) women have during labour and their opinions
about them.

We are sending this questionnaire to women who have had babies in the
hospital since 1978.   We would be very grateful if you would be kind
enough to fill in this questionnaire on both sides and send it back in
the envelope supplied (it does not need a stamp).   This information will
be kept confidential and will only be used for research, with no names attached.

It is very important that you return the questionnaire, even if you have had
no health problems, so that we can get an overall picture which takes everyone
into account.   We are sure you realise that the information you give will
help us to provide better care for all new mothers-to-be coming to this hospital.

Thank you in advance for all your time and help.

Yours sincerely,

J. Selwyn Crawford, FFARCS., FRCOG
M. Lewis, FFARCS.

Consultant Anaesthetists

Encl.

Central Birmingham Health Authority

Appendix 2

In this Appendix, which will be used chiefly for reference purposes, we relate each of the factors included in the study to all of the others. The purpose of this exercise is to indicate the extremely complex nature of the relationships between all of the social, obstetric and anaesthetic factors. Taking account of such inter-relationships is crucial in our attempt to distinguish primary from secondary associations in identifying any potential determinants of the various health problems.

The first comparison we give is for parity (Table A.1). This table compares primiparous with multiparous women with respect to each of the other variables. On the first line we compare maternal age, showing that 37.2% of the parity 0 women were under 25 years compared with only 14.2% of the parity 1+ women. The second line gives a comparison of marital status according to parity, then social class and so on. This is the format we have followed in all the Tables shown in this Appendix.

Parity. Table A.1 compares women having their first child with those delivering a subsequent child. Parity was associated with almost every other factor. Women having their first babies were more likely to be younger, unmarried, from lower social classes, shorter and Afro-Caribbean. Inductions, atypical presentations and raised blood pressure were all more frequent, and both stages of labour (especially second) were much longer. Forceps deliveries and emergency sections were much more frequent, as were post-partum haemorrhages and episiotomies, but not lacerations. All types of analgesia and anaesthesia, except for inhalation, were used more often by primiparous women. First babies were more likely to be pre-term, smaller, admitted to special care and breast fed.

Maternal age. Table A.2 also shows a wide range of associations. Younger women were more likely to be primiparous, unmarried or from social classes III, IV and V. They were more likely to be Asian or Afro-Caribbean than Caucasian. Twins and hypertension were less frequent among younger women and long labours were a little more frequent. Pain relief patterns differed between maternal age-bands but not as much as for parity: the same applied to gestation and infant size at delivery. Breast feeding was more frequent in older women. Many of the relationships between maternal age and the obstetric and anaesthetic factors are probably indirect, and secondary to the strong associations with primiparity.

Marital status. This was associated with fewer factors (Table A.3). The main associations were that unmarried women were much more likely to be having their first baby, to be under 25 years of age, of lower social class and

TABLE A.1

Factors	Parity 0 (n = 4185) %	Parity 1+ (n = 7516) %	
Primiparous	–	–	
Under 25 years	37.2	14.2	
Married	83.2	93.7	
Social class I, II	22.3	25.9	
Caucasian	86.5	86.7	
Asian	4.7	4.5	NS
Afro-Caribbean	4.2	2.8	
Under 160 cms tall	33.5	34.6	
Hypertension	12.4	7.1	
Ante-partum haemorrhage	3.1	2.6	NS
Induced labour	14.9	10.8	
Occipito-anterior	84.9	89.4	
Multiple pregnancy	1.6	1.4	NS
1st stage 6 hrs or more	31.0	10.6	
2nd stage 1 hr or more	55.3	14.0	
Forceps	36.4	10.3	
Elective section	3.8	8.1	
Emergency section	15.1	6.8	
Episiotomy	61.3	33.9	
Laceration	14.1	30.9	
Post-partum haemorrhage	17.1	10.2	
Epidural	55.6	32.4	
Pethidine	20.7	10.5	
Inhalation	40.0	43.1	
Tranquillisers	7.8	4.6	
Pudendal block	4.5	1.3	
Spinal block	2.2	0.9	
General anaesthetic	11.2	9.2	
No analgesia or anaesthesia	3.3	13.7	
Pre-term	8.0	6.2	
Low birthweight (up to 2500 grams)	8.1	5.7	
Head circ. 32 cms or less	14.2	9.6	
Length 47 cms or less	12.7	10.7	
Special care	11.9	8.8	
Breast feeding	73.3	64.8	

TABLE A.2

Factors	Maternal age			
	Under 25 yrs (n = 2625)	25-29 yrs (n = 4225)	30 yrs or more (n = 4851)	
Primiparous	59.4	36.1	22.7	
Under 25 years	–	–	–	
Married	72.2	94.4	95.7	
Social class I, II	6.4	23.8	35.2	
Caucasian	80.9	88.6	88.0	
Asian	7.8	4.0	3.2	
Afro-Caribbean	7.6	2.8	1.4	
Under 160 cms tall	39.2	34.3	31.5	
Hypertension	7.7	8.3	10.3	
Ante-partum haemorrhage	2.5	1.9	3.7	
Induced labour	11.7	11.7	13.1	
Occipito-anterior	88.3	88.4	87.0	NS
Multiple pregnancy	0.7	1.7	1.6	
1st stage 6 hrs or more	26.7	23.1	18.9	
2nd stage 1 hr or more	33.2	29.1	24.9	
Forceps	21.6	20.6	17.8	
Elective section	3.1	5.6	9.3	
Emergency section	9.6	8.9	10.7	
Episiotomy	45.6	45.3	41.2	
Laceration	22.9	26.2	24.8	
Post-partum haemorrhage	13.0	12.2	13.0	NS
Epidural	42.1	40.0	40.6	NS
Pethidine	20.1	14.8	10.4	
Inhalation	45.3	44.4	38.1	
Tranquillisers	7.4	6.3	4.4	
Pudendal block	2.5	2.8	2.1	
Spinal block	1.6	1.4	1.2	NS
General anaesthetic	8.0	8.4	12.2	
No analgesia or anaesthesia	8.4	9.8	11.0	
Pre-term	7.6	6.1	7.1	
Low birthweight (up to 2500 grams)	6.7	5.9	7.0	
Head circ. 32 cms or less	13.9	10.7	10.3	
Length 47 cms or less	12.3	11.0	11.3	
Special care	9.8	8.7	11.0	
Breast feeding	57.7	70.2	71.2	

TABLE A.3

Factors	Married (n = 10525) %	Not married (n = 1176) %	
Primiparous	33.1	59.7	
Under 25 years	18.0	62.2	
Married	–	–	
Social class I, II	26.9	4.0	
Caucasian	87.8	75.8	
Asian	4.9	0.9	
Afro-Caribbean	1.5	19.2	
Under 160 cms tall	34.2	34.4	NS
Hypertension	9.3	6.9	
Ante-partum haemorrhage	2.8	2.5	NS
Induced labour	12.4	11.2	NS
Occipito-anterior	87.8	87.2	NS
Multiple pregnancy	1.5	0.9	NS
1st stage 6 hrs or more	22.5	27.7	
2nd stage 1 hr or more	28.3	29.2	NS
Forceps	19.7	19.0	NS
Elective section	6.9	3.3	
Emergency section	9.7	10.5	NS
Episiotomy	43.9	41.7	NS
Laceration	25.4	19.7	
Post-partum haemorrhage	12.7	12.9	NS
Epidural	40.7	40.7	NS
Pethidine	13.6	19.0	
Inhalation	41.7	44.9	
Tranquillisers	5.7	6.2	NS
Pudendal block	2.5	1.8	NS
Spinal block	1.4	1.4	NS
General anaesthetic	10.0	8.9	NS
No analgesia or anaesthesia	10.1	9.3	NS
Pre-term	6.7	8.3	
Low birthweight (up to 2500 grams)	6.3	8.8	
Head circ. 32 cms or less	10.8	15.6	
Length 47 cms or less	11.1	14.5	
Special care	9.7	11.2	NS
Breast feeding	68.8	58.8	

Afro-Caribbean. In obstetric terms, married women were more likely to have had hypertension, an elective section and a bigger baby. Breast feeding was also associated with being married.

Social class. The social class distribution is given in Table A.4 – unmarried women or those whose husbands were students or whose occupation was not known, have been excluded. The biggest social class difference was for maternal age: women in social classes III, IV and V tended to be younger. Hypertension was more likely among social classes III, IV and V. Small babies were more frequent, breast feeding at discharge less frequent and there was an increased usage of Pethidine, inhalation analgesia and tranquillisers, with epidural anaesthesia being less common.

Ethnic group. Table A.5 compares Caucasian, Asian and Afro-Caribbean women. There were substantial differences. The Asian women in this population resembled the Caucasians in their parity and social class distributions but they were younger, shorter and a higher proportion were married. They had fewer induced labours, less hypertension, shorter second stage labours and more emergency sections. Their babies were more likely to be smaller and admitted to the Special Care Baby Unit.

The Afro-Caribbean women were more often primiparous, younger, of lower social class, and as many as 58% were unmarried. They had less hypertension and fewer induced labours. The forceps rate was much lower even though a higher proportion were primiparous, but there were more emergency sections. The second stage of labour was much shorter with durations in excess of one hour occurring only half as often as among Caucasian women. Afro-Caribbean women used far fewer epidurals and much more pethidine and inhalation analgesia. The babies were smaller (although not pre-term) and more often admitted to the Special Care Baby Unit. Breast feeding was much more frequent.

Maternal height. Table A.6 shows that short stature was closely associated with lower social class and Asian ethnic origins. Shorter women had more elective and emergency sections; among women under 160 cms in height, 21.1% had a section compared with 9.1% in women of 170 cms or more. Increased infant birthweight, head circumference and length were associated with increased maternal height.

Hypertension. Table A.7 shows that women who had hypertension were much more likely to be primiparous. Women aged 25 years or more, married, lower social class and Caucasian were also a little more likely to have hypertension. Hypertension was associated with induced labour (39%) and with longer second stage labours, forceps delivery, emergency and elective sections, and post-partum haemorrhage. Epidural anaesthesia was more frequently used in

TABLE A.4

Factors	Social class*		
	I and II (n = 2882) %	III, IV, V (n = 7048) %	
Primiparous	32.4	33.6	NS**
Under 25 years	5.8	20.8	
Married	N/A	N/A	
Social class I, II	—	—	
Caucasian	86.7	89.1	
Asian	3.5	4.5	
Afro-Caribbean	1.3	1.8	
Under 160 cms tall	27.7	35.8	
Hypertension	8.1	10.1	
Ante-partum haemorrhage	2.5	2.8	NS
Induced labour	12.3	12.5	NS
Occipito-anterior	87.5	88.0	NS
Multiple pregnancy	1.6	1.5	NS
1st stage 6 hrs or more	22.2	21.8	NS
2nd stage 1 hr or more	27.3	29.0	NS
Forceps	20.9	19.4	NS
Elective section	8.8	6.2	
Emergency section	8.8	10.0	
Episiotomy	46.3	43.9	
Laceration	26.0	25.2	NS
Post-partum haemorrhage	11.7	13.0	NS
Epidural	42.6	40.3	
Pethidine	10.9	14.6	
Inhalation	38.7	42.5	
Tranquillisers	4.9	6.2	
Pudendal block	2.5	2.5	NS
Spinal block	1.2	1.4	NS
General anaesthetic	10.1	9.9	NS
No analgesia or anaesthesia	10.5	9.9	NS
Pre-term	6.5	6.4	NS
Low birthweight (up to 2500 grams)	5.2	6.4	
Head circ. 32 cms or less	9.0	11.1	
Length 47 cms or less	10.2	11.4	
Special care	8.9	9.8	NS
Breast feeding	83.6	64.4	

*Unclassified are excluded

**There was a difference at higher parities with social class III, IV, V, delivering more 4th or subsequent children.

TABLE A.5

	Ethnic group		
Factors	**Caucasian** **(n = 10135)**	**Asian** **(n = 530)**	**Afro Caribbean*** **(n = 388)**	
Primiparous	35.7	36.8	44.8	
Under 25 years	20.9	38.5	51.3	
Married	91.2	97.9	41.8	
Social class I, II	24.7	19.1	9.8	
Caucasian	–	–	–	
Asian	–	–	–	
Afro-Caribbean	–	–	–	
Under 160 cms tall	33.0	65.1	31.7	
Hypertension	9.3	5.5	4.4	
Ante-partum haemorrhage	2.8	2.6	3.6	NS
Induced labour	12.6	7.5	7.0	
Occipito-anterior	87.8	87.9	90.2	NS
Multiple pregnancy	1.5	0.9	1.0	NS
1st stage 6 hrs or more	22.5	27.4	24.0	
2nd stage 1 hr or more	29.2	21.1	15.2	
Forceps	20.0	19.4	9.0	
Elective section	6.5	6.0	4.4	
Emergency section	9.5	13.6	12.1	
Episiotomy	43.9	37.9	27.1	
Laceration	25.6	24.3	23.5	
Post-partum haemorrhage	12.9	13.6	15.7	NS
Epidural	41.1	38.1	27.6	
Pethidine	13.6	18.5	22.7	
Inhalation	42.6	40.0	52.6	
Tranquillisers	5.5	5.1	5.7	NS
Pudendal block	2.6	1.7	1.0	
Spinal block	1.4	1.9	1.0	NS
General anaesthetic	9.2	14.3	12.6	
No analgesia or anaesthesia	10.0	10.2	11.9	NS
Pre-term	6.7	8.1	8.2	NS
Low birthweight (up to 2500 grams)	6.1	9.8	11.6	
Head circ. 32 cms or less	10.3	19.8	21.9	
Length 47 cms or less	10.9	16.4	18.3	
Special care	9.5	11.1	11.1	
Breast feeding	67.2	62.5	88.4	

*Other races excluded

TABLE A.6

Maternal heights*

Factors

	Under 160 cms (n = 4004)	160-169 cms (n = 5829)	170 cms or more (n = 1105)	
Primiparous	35.0	36.1	41.4	
Under 25 years	25.7	21.5	18.0	
Married	89.9	89.6	91.5	NS
Social class I, II	19.9	25.2	33.2	
Caucasian	83.6	89.5	90.9	
Asian	8.6	2.6	0.7	
Afro-Caribbean	3.1	3.5	3.3	
Under 160 cms tall	–	–	–	
Hypertension	8.5	9.0	10.0	NS
Ante-partum haemorrhage	3.0	2.7	2.3	NS
Induced labour	11.0	12.5	15.8	
Occipito-anterior	87.4	88.2	88.7	NS
Multiple pregnancy	1.2	1.3	2.2	
1st stage 6 hrs or more	23.3	21.4	23.7	NS
2nd stage 1 hr or more	27.8	29.2	30.2	NS
Forceps	18.6	20.3	21.4	
Elective section	8.6	5.2	3.3	
Emergency section	12.5	8.1	5.8	
Episiotomy	41.2	45.2	46.4	
Laceration	22.5	26.3	28.9	
Post-partum haemorrhage	13.2	12.4	12.9	NS
Epidural	41.9	39.9	40.3	NS
Pethidine	14.6	14.3	15.1	NS
Inhalation	40.1	43.9	44.4	
Tranquillisers	5.6	6.0	5.7	NS
Pudendal block	2.1	2.6	3.3	NS
Spinal block	1.4	1.2	2.2	NS
General anaesthetic	12.7	7.7	5.1	
No analgesia or anaesthesia	9.2	10.1	11.9	
Pre-term	6.4	5.6	5.0	
Low birthweight (up to 2500 grams)	7.1	5.1	3.3	
Head circ. 32 cms or less	13.7	9.1	5.3	
Length 47 cms or less	9.4	7.3	5.4	
Special care	9.6	8.6	7.1	
Breast feeding	62.7	70.1	78.9	

*Those 763 women for whom height was not recorded are excluded from this Table

TABLE A.7

Maternal hypertension

Factors	Hypertension (n = 1055) %	No hypertension (n = 10646) %	
Primiparous	49.4	34.4	
Under 25 years	19.2	22.8	
Married	92.3	89.7	
Social class I, II	22.1	24.9	
Caucasian	88.9	86.4	
Asian	2.7	4.7	
Afro-Caribbean	1.6	3.5	
Under 160 cms tall	32.3	34.4	NS
Hypertension	−	−	
Ante-partum haemorrhage	2.1	2.9	NS
Induced labour	39.1	9.6	
Occipito-anterior	81.8	88.4	
Multiple pregnancy	3.0	1.3	
1st stage 6 hrs or more	24.3	23.0	
2nd stage 1 hr or more	40.0	27.5	
Forceps	26.5	19.0	
Elective section	10.4	6.2	
Emergency section	19.9	8.8	
Episiotomy	43.3	43.7	NS
Laceration	16.6	25.7	
Post-partum haemorrhage	18.7	12.1	
Epidural	58.1	39.0	
Pethidine	9.0	14.7	
Inhalation	26.2	43.6	
Tranquillisers	5.8	5.7	NS
Pudendal block	2.5	2.4	NS
Spinal block	1.0	1.4	NS
General anaesthetic	19.4	9.0	
No analgesia or anaesthesia	3.9	10.6	
Pre-term	13.3	6.2	
Low birthweight (up to 2500 grams)	15.3	5.7	
Head circ. 32 cms or less	15.9	10.8	
Length 47 cms or less	18.6	10.7	
Special care	21.0	8.8	
Breast feeding	64.1	68.2	

association with hypertension and the infants were much more likely to be pre-term and of low birthweight.

Ante-partum haemorrhage. Table A.8 groups all types of ante-partum haemorrhage together and shows that this was associated with induction of labour, Caesarean section – particularly emergency section (RR = 3.1) – and, probably as a consequence of Caesarean section, with post-partum haemorrhage. Ante-partum haemorrhage was also associated with pre-term deliveries, with smaller babies and with more frequent admission to special care.

Onset of labour. Table A.9 shows that induced labour was associated with first babies, with multiple pregnancy and with maternal hypertension – the latter accounted for more than a quarter of all induced labours. Inductions were less frequent among Asian and Afro-Caribbean women. Induction was associated with prolonged second stage of labour, but not first stage. Forceps and emergency sections were more frequent as was usage of epidural anaesthesia. Large babies with large heads were more likely to be induced, and admission to special care was more frequent. (Elective sections have been excluded from these comparisons).

Fetal presentation. Table A.10 shows that only one maternal characteristic was associated with atypical fetal presentations: they were more frequent in primiparous women. Atypical presentations however were associated with numerous obstetric factors: with maternal hypertension, ante-partum haemorrhage, longer labour (especially second stage) and Caesarean sections – particularly emergency sections (RR = 4.9). Correspondingly, post-partum haemorrhage was more common. Epidural and spinal anaesthesia and pudendal blocks were also more frequent with atypical presentations. Deliveries were more likely to be pre-term, babies were smaller and more likely to be admitted to special care.

Multiple pregnancy. Table A.11 demonstrates the associations of multiple pregnancy. All but six of the 169 multiple pregnancies in this population were twins, the remainder triplets. Women who delivered more than one baby were less likely to be under 25 years, but there were no other associations with maternal characteristics. Not surprisingly there were many differences in obstetric and anaesthetic characteristics. There were higher rates of hypertension, long labours (especially second stage), emergency (but not elective) sections and post-partum haemorrhage among women with multiple deliveries. Epidural anaesthesia was much more often used as pain relief. Pre-term deliveries were much more frequent than for singletons (RR = 7.0) and admission to special care was more likely (RR = 6.2) Twins were much less likely to be breast fed.

TABLE A.8

Ante-partum haemorrhage

Factors	APH (n = 327) %	No APH (n = 11374) %	
Primiparous	39.1	35.7	NS
Under 25 years	20.2	22.5*	
Married	91.1	89.9	NS
Social class I, II	22.0	24.7	NS
Caucasian	85.3	86.7	NS
Asian	4.3	4.5	NS
Afro-Caribbean	4.3	3.3	NS
Under 160 cms tall	37.0	34.1	NS
Hypertension	6.7	9.1	NS
Ante-partum haemorrhage	−	−	
Induced labour	19.0	12.1	
Occipito-anterior	82.6	87.9	
Multiple pregnancy	2.4	1.4	NS
1st stage 6 hrs or more	24.4	22.2	NS
2nd stage 1 hr or more	19.3	24.0	NS
Forceps	18.3	19.7	NS
Elective section	12.8	6.4	
Emergency section	28.4	9.2	
Episiotomy	34.3	44.0	
Laceration	14.1	25.2	
Post-partum haemorrhage	27.2	12.3	
Epidural	39.1	40.8	NS
Pethidine	8.0	14.3	
Inhalation	24.8	42.5	
Tranquillisers	3.4	5.8	NS
Pudendal block	1.5	2.5	NS
Spinal block	0.6	1.4	NS
General anaesthetic	34.9	9.2	
No analgesia or anaesthesia	5.5	10.1	
Pre-term	26.9	6.3	
Low birthweight (up to 2500 grams)	23.2	6.1	
Head circ. 32 cms or less	27.5	10.8	
Length 47 cms or less	23.9	11.1	
Special care	28.4	9.3	
Breast feeding	59.6	68.1	

*This is significant using T-test with over 30's more APH's

TABLE A.9

Type of onset of labour*

Factors	Induced (n = 1434) %	Spontaneous (n = 9497) %	
Primiparous	43.2	35.9	
Under 25 years	21.4	23.6	
Married	90.8	89.4	NS
Social class I, II	24.7	23.9	NS
Caucasian	89.3	86.3	
Asian	2.7	4.8	
Afro-Caribbean	1.9	3.6	
Under 160 cms tall	30.7	33.9	
Hypertension	28.8	5.6	
Ante-partum haemorrhage	4.3	2.3	
Induced labour	–	–	
Occipito-anterior	87.4	88.8	NS
Multiple pregnancy	2.4	1.3	
1st stage 6 hrs or more	20.3	22.6	
2nd stage 1 hr or more	37.9	24.5	
Forceps	29.1	19.8	
Elective section	N/A	N/A	
Emergency section	14.2	9.9	
Episiotomy	51.3	46.1	
Laceration	20.9	27.4	
Post-partum haemorrhage	14.1	10.6	
Epidural	65.6	35.8	
Pethidine	15.7	15.0	NS
Inhalation	29.4	47.3	
Tranquillisers	6.4	6.1	NS
Pudendal block	2.6	2.6	NS
Spinal block	1.3	1.5	NS
General anaesthetic	8.1	7.2	NS
No analgesia or anaesthesia	3.5	11.8	
Pre-term	4.5	6.9	
Low birthweight (up to 2500 grams)	5.6	6.4**	
Head circ. 32 cms or less	8.9	11.7	
Length 47 cms or less	9.8	11.2	
Special care	12.6	8.6	
Breast feeding	64.6	68.9	

*Elective sections (n = 770) are excluded

**There was a statistical association with birthweight in its continuous format using a T-test, the main feature being that induced onset was associated with very big babies.

TABLE A.10

Type of fetal presentation

Factors	Occipito-anterior (n = 10271) %	Atypical (n = 1430) %	
Primiparous	34.6	44.1	
Under 25 years	22.6	21.5	NS
Married	90.0	89.4	NS
Social class I, II	24.6	25.3	NS
Caucasian	86.6	86.6	NS
Asian	4.5	4.5	NS
Afro-Caribbean	3.4	2.7	NS
Under 160 cms tall	34.1	35.2	NS
Hypertension	8.4	13.4	
Ante-partum haemorrhage	2.6	4.0	
Induced labour	12.2	12.7	NS
Occipito-anterior	−	−	
Multiple pregnancy	N/A	N/A	
1st stage 6 hrs or more	22.6	28.2	
2nd stage 1 hr or more	27.4	40.0	
Forceps	19.6	20.4*	NS
Elective section	5.6	13.6	
Emergency section	6.6	32.5	
Episiotomy	43.6	44.0	NS
Laceration	27.4	6.6	
Post-partum haemorrhage	10.8	26.4	
Epidural	38.2	59.0	
Pethidine	14.8	9.8	
Inhalation	44.4	24.5	
Tranquillisers	5.9	4.4	
Pudendal block	2.2	8.8	
Spinal block	1.2	2.4	
General anaesthetic	7.5	26.8	
No analgesia or anaesthesia	10.9	3.6	
Pre-term	5.8	14.1	
Low birthweight (up to 2500 grams)	5.4	14.9	
Head circ. 32 cms or less	10.6	15.8	
Length 47 cms or less	10.6	17.3	
Special care	8.5	19.9	
Breast feeding	68.4	63.8	

*There was a significant difference between atypical presentations and rotational forceps.

TABLE A.11

Multiple pregnancy

Factors	Multiple (n = 169) %	Singleton (n = 11532) %	
Primiparous	38.5	35.7	NS
Under 25 years	11.2	22.6	
Married	94.1	89.9	NS
Social class I, II	1.6	1.5	NS
Caucasian	87.0	86.6	NS
Asian	3.0	4.6	NS
Afro-Caribbean	2.4	3.8	NS
Under 160 cms tall	27.8	34.3	
Hypertension	18.9	8.9	
Ante-partum haemorrhage	4.7	2.8	
Induced labour	20.7	12.2	
Occipito-anterior	N/A	N/A	
Multiple pregnancy	–	–	
1st stage 6 hrs or more	26.9	23.0	NS
2nd stage 1 hr or more	41.9	28.2	
Forceps	N/A	N/A	
Elective section	7.1	6.6	NS
Emergency section	23.7	9.6	
Episiotomy	53.3	43.5	
Laceration	9.5	25.1	
Post-partum haemorrhage	30.8	12.4	
Epidural	65.7	40.4	
Pethidine	4.1	14.3	
Inhalation	23.7	42.3	
Tranquillisers	3.6	5.8	NS
Pudendal block	3.6	2.4	NS
Spinal block	0.6	1.4	NS
General anaesthetic	22.5	9.7	
No analgesia or anaesthesia	1.8	10.1	
Pre-term	44.4	6.3	
Low birthweight (up to 2500 grams)	N/A	N/A	
Head circ. 32 cms or less	N/A	N/A	
Length 47 cms or less	N/A	N/A	
Special care	56.8	9.2	
Breast feeding	46.7	68.1	

Duration of labour. The duration of first (Table A.12) and second (Table A.13) stages of labour were very closely inter-related, with a short first stage beig much more frequently followed by a short second stage. Duration of labour, both stages, was also highly associated with many maternal, obstetric and anaesthetic characteristics. Primiparous women had much longer labours, both stages, as did younger women. Asian women were a little more likely to have a longer first stage and Afro-Caribbean were much more likely to have a short second stage. Induced labours had longer second stages. Forceps deliveries were closely associated with longer labours, particularly second stage, such that a women who had a second stage of one hour or more was 12.7 times as likely to have a forceps delivery as a women with a second stage of 15 minutes or less. Episiotomy was also much more common in association with a long labour, especially second stage. Epidural and spinal anaesthesia were both highly associated with longer labour, particularly second; 72.8% of women with a second stage of one hour or more had an epidural, compared with only 11.9% of those with a second stage of 15 minutes or less. A longer labour was also associated with a bigger baby.

Forceps (Table A.14). Most of the forceps used in this population were the non-rotational type. Since the two main types of forceps differ greatly we have compared them separately. Both rotational and non-rotational forceps were much more frequent among primiparous women; both were less often used for Afro-Caribbean women. Both types of forceps were associated with induced labours, longer labours, especially second stage, and episiotomies. Rotational forceps only were closely associated with an atypical fetal presentation and with a post-partum haemorrhage. Epidural anaesthesia was closely associated with both types of forceps: pudendal block was more common with non-rotational forceps and a spinal block with rotational forceps. Babies delivered by forceps were more likely to be bigger.

Caesarean section (Table A.15). We compared the two different types of section, elective and emergency, with vaginal deliveries. Associations here were found in relation to every other factor. Primiparous and younger women were more likely to have an emergency section. Shorter women were more likely to have either type of section as were women with hypertension. Atypical fetal presentations occurred in association with 40.7% of the emergency sections and 25.3% of elective sections, compared with only 7.9% of vaginal deliveries. Epidural anaesthesia was more common in association with both types of section than vaginal delivery and so was a post-partum haemorrhage. Babies delivered by either types of section were more likely to be pre-term and smaller but this was especially so for emergency sections. They were also much more likely to be admitted to special care.

TABLE A.12

Duration of first stage of labour*

Factors

	Under 2 hrs (n = 2055)	2 hrs – 5 hrs 59 mins (n = 5264)	6 hours or more (n = 2195)	
Primiparous	15.0	33.1	59.1	
Under 25 years	18.6	23.3	28.1	
Married	91.5	89.9	87.7	
Social class I, II	24.1	24.4	24.1	NS
Caucasian	89.5	87.2	85.0	
Asian	3.7	4.2	5.1	
Afro-Caribbean	3.1	3.3	3.4	NS
Under 160 cms tall	33.7	31.4	33.8	NS
Hypertension	6.6	9.7	8.0	NS
Ante-partum haemorrhage	1.8	2.0	2.1	NS
Induced labour	11.0	14.2	11.5	
Occipito-anterior	94.1	91.9	90.2	
Multiple pregnancy	1.0	1.3	1.5	NS
1st stage 6 hrs or more	–	–	–	
2nd stage 1 hr or more	90.9	80.0	49.3	
Forceps	8.8	21.3	42.6	
Elective section	N/A	N/A	N/A	
Emergency section	N/A	N/A	N/A	
Episiotomy	37.5	51.1	67.7	
Laceration	36.6	31.2	19.2	
Post-partum haemorrhage	3.9	7.0	11.3	
Epidural	16.3	38.2	60.6	
Pethidine	11.5	16.5	19.6	
Inhalation	54.2	49.4	42.2	
Tranquillisers	4.3	6.9	7.7	
Pudendal block	2.0	2.9	3.3	
Spinal block	1.1	1.6	1.7	
General anaesthetic	N/A	N/A	N/A	
No analgesia or anaesthesia	20.4	10.4	4.7	
Pre-term	5.4	4.9	4.1	
Low birthweight (up to 2500 grams)	5.5	4.6	3.5	
Head circ. 32 cms or less	11.0	10.6	7.8	
Length 47 cms or less	11.2	9.6	8.5	
Special care	6.9	6.5	6.9	NS
Breast feeding	68.3	69.0	71.3	NS

*Caesarean sections and those women where duration was not recorded, are excluded.

TABLE A.13

Duration of second stage of labour*

Factors

	Up to 15 mins (n = 3015) %	16 mins – 59 mins (n = 3891) %	One hour or more (n = 2797) %	
Primiparous	7.4	32.6	68.0	
Under 25 years	18.7	24.3	27.4	
Married	90.1	89.4	89.3	NS
Social class I, II	22.8	25.8	23.2	NS
Caucasian	86.2	86.1	89.7	
Asian	4.2	4.3	4.6	NS
Afro-Caribbean	4.6	3.3	1.8	
Under 160 cms tall	33.0	32.4	31.6	NS
Hypertension	5.0	7.2	10.6	
Ante-partum haemorrhage	1.8	1.9	2.3	NS
Induced labour	9.5	12.2	16.9	
Occipito-anterior	95.9	91.3	88.5	
Multiple pregnancy	0.3	1.5	1.9	
1st stage 6 hrs or more	11.3	19.0	39.5	
2nd stage 1 hr or more	–	–	–	
Forceps	4.4	14.3	55.9	
Elective section	N/A	N/A	N/A	
Emergency section	N/A	N/A	N/A	
Episiotomy	25.5	52.8	74.2	
Laceration	42.0	30.8	14.5	
Post-partum haemorrhage	3.7	5.7	13.2	
Epidural	11.9	33.4	72.8	
Pethidine	14.5	17.4	15.7	NS
Inhalation	58.4	50.4	35.8	
Tranquillisers	5.5	8.0	5.4	
Pudendal block	0.8	2.7	5.3	
Spinal block	0.4	1.1	3.3	
General anaesthetic	N/A	N/A	N/A	
No analgesia or anaesthesia	21.4	10.8	2.4	
Pre-term	5.0	5.4	4.1	NS
Low birthweight (up to 2500 grams)	4.7	5.7	2.9	
Head circ. 32 cms or less	11.2	10.9	7.9	
Length 47 cms or less	11.1	10.2	7.6	
Special care	6.5	7.6	5.8	NS
Breast feeding	68.0	69.7	70.4	NS

*Caesarean sections and those women where duration was not recorded, are excluded.

TABLE A.14

Forceps deliveries

Factors

	Non-rotational forceps (n = 1858) %	Rotational forceps (n = 443) %	No forceps (n = 9400) %	
Primiparous	65.8	68.2	28.3	
Under 25 years	25.0	23.3	21.9	
Married	90.4	89.8	89.9	NS
Social class I, II	25.9	26.9	24.3	NS
Caucasian	88.2	87.8	86.2	
Asian	4.2	5.6	4.5	NS
Afro-Caribbean	1.6	1.1	3.8	
Under 160 cms tall	31.0	38.1	34.7	
Hypertension	11.6	14.7	8.2	
Ante-partum haemorrhage	2.6	2.5	2.8	NS
Induced labour	17.4	21.0	10.8	
Occipito-anterior	92.4	65.9	87.8	
Multiple pregnancy	N/A	N/A	N/A	
1st stage 6 hrs or more	40.8	41.1	16.7	
2nd stage 1 hr or more	69.4	71.8	16.3	
Forceps	—	—	—	
Elective section	N/A	N/A	N/A	
Emergency section	N/A	N/A	N/A	
Episiotomy	96.0	98.2	30.8	
Laceration	3.3	2.9	30.1	
Post-partum haemorrhage	14.2	17.4	12.2	
Epidural	77.3	85.3	31.4	
Pethidine	13.7	11.5	14.4	NS
Inhalation	33.2	24.6	44.6	
Tranquillisers	5.0	4.5	6.0	
Pudendal block	11.3	3.6	0.6	
Spinal block	3.3	9.7	0.6	
General anaesthetic	0.9	1.1	12.1	
No analgesia or anaesthesia	0.4	—	12.4	
Pre-term	5.4	3.2	7.3	
Low birthweight (up to 2500 grams)	4.7	2.0	7.1	
Head circ. 32 cms or less	8.9	7.4	11.9	
Length 47 cms or less	8.7	7.2	12.2	
Special care	8.3	5.4	10.4	
Breast feeding	69.1	72.5	67.4	

TABLE A.15

Caesarean section

Factors

	Emergency (n = 1145) %	Elective (n = 770) %	Vaginal (n = 9786) %
Primiparous	55.2	20.5	34.7
Under 25 years	21.9	10.5	23.4
Married	89.2	94.9	89.6
Social class I, II	22.1	33.0	24.3
Caucasian	83.8	85.3	87.0
Asian	6.3	4.2	4.4
Afro-Caribbean	4.1	2.2	3.3
Under 160 cms tall	43.8	44.9	32.3
Hypertension	18.3	14.3	7.5
Ante-partum haemorrhage	8.1	5.5	2.0
Induced labour	17.7	N/A	12.6
Occipito-anterior	59.3	74.7	92.1
Multiple pregnancy	3.5	1.6	1.2
1st stage 6 hrs or more	N/A	N/A	N/A
2nd stage 1 hr or more	N/A	N/A	N/A
Forceps	N/A	N/A	N/A
Elective section	–	–	–
Emergency section	–	–	–
Episiotomy	N/A	N/A	N/A
Laceration	N/A	N/A	N/A
Post-partum haemorrhage	45.1	36.2	7.1
Epidural	56.9	55.3	37.7
Pethidine	8.5	0.5	15.9
Inhalation	14.1	0.4	48.5
Tranquillisers	3.6	0.1	6.4
Pudendal block	0.2	–	2.9
Spinal block	0.9	–	1.5
General anaesthetic	65.8	47.0	0.4
No analgesia or anaesthesia	N/A	N/A	N/A
Pre-term	20.0	10.8	5.0
Low birthweight (up to 2500 grams)	20.3	10.6	4.6
Head circ. 32 cms or less	21.0	10.1	10.2
Length 47 cms or less	21.0	17.7	9.8
Special care	29.8	20.1	6.7
Breast feeding	59.6	61.0	69.3

Perineal complications (Table A.16) include both episiotomy and laceration, these being compared with each other and with an intact perineum. This table includes all deliveries; many of the women with an intact perineum will have had a Caesarean section. Some major differences were shown. Episiotomies were much more frequently given to primiparous women, whilst multiparae were equally likely to have either laceration or an intact perineum. Atypical fetal presentations were closely associated with either episiotomy or an intact perineum, the latter because of the high section rate amongst this group. Longer labours and forceps deliveries were both associated with episiotomy. Epidural and spinal anaesthesia were also positively associated with episiotomy, whilst inhalation was associated with perineal tears.

Post-partum haemorrhage (PPH) (Table A.17). This was more frequent among primiparous women but was not associated with any of the other maternal characteristics. Over half of the PPH's were recorded in association with Caesarean sections. A PPH was also associated with a long second stage labour. In durations of two hours or more the relative risk of a PPH was 5.0 compared with durations of 15 minutes or less. Women who had a PPH were more likely to deliver babies that were pre-term and smaller, these associations probably resulting directly from the association with Caesarean section.

Types of analgesia and anaesthesia (Tables A.18-A.24). The various types of analgesia and anaesthesia experienced by the women were closely inter-related since having one type would often preclude the likelihood or necessity of having another type. Primiparous women were more likely to have had some form of analgesia or anaesthesia than multiparous women. In general, epidural anaesthesia was closely associated with maternal hypertension, induced labour, multiple pregnancy, atypical fetal presentation, long labour, forceps, section, episiotomy and post-partum haemorrhage. Inhalation, the other most frequently used type of analgesia, was associated with occipito-anterior fetal presentation, short labour, normal deliveries and perineal tears. There was no large or striking differences for pethidine usage. It was a little more common among younger women and those in social classes III, IV and V. Tranquillisers were not frequently used, but were a little more common among younger women, lower social class women and where the first stage of labour was long. Pudendal block was highly associated with a forceps delivery, atypical fetal presentation, long labour and episiotomy. Spinal anaesthesia was similarly associated with atypical fetal presentation, long second stage labour, forceps delivery and episiotomy: only 10 women had a section using this form of anaesthesia. General anaesthesia not surprisingly was rarely given for anything but Caesarean section so that its associations mirrored closely those already described for Caesarean section.

TABLE A.16

Perineal complications at delivery

Factors

	Episiotomy* (n = 5112) %	Laceration* (n = 2907) %	Intact** (n = 3749) %
Primiparous	50.2	20.2	22.5
Under 25 years	23.4	25.8	21.8
Married	90.4	92.0	87.8
Social class I, II	26.1	20.6	21.8
Caucasian	87.1	89.3	84.1
Asian	3.9	4.4	5.4
Afro-Caribbean	2.1	3.1	5.1
Under 160 cms tall	32.3	31.0	39.3
Hypertension	8.9	6.0	11.4
Ante-partum haemorrhage	2.2	1.6	4.6
Induced labour	14.4	10.3	11.0
Occipito-anterior	87.7	96.7	80.8
Multiple pregnancy	1.8	0.6	1.7
1st stage 6 hrs or more	30.1	15.0	15.7
2nd stage 1 hr or more	43.3	14.0	10.9
Forceps	43.4	2.5	1.1
Elective section	N/A	N/A	N/A
Emergency section	N/A	N/A	N/A
Episiotomy	–	–	–
Laceration	–	–	–
Post-partum haemorrhage	9.7	9.8	22.9
Epidural	52.9	22.0	38.7
Pethidine	16.9	14.9	10.2
Inhalation	42.5	57.0	30.1
Tranquillisers	7.5	4.6	4.3
Pudendal block	5.3	0.5	0.2
Spinal block	2.5	0.8	0.5
General anaesthetic	0.7	0.2	29.6
No analgesia or anaesthesia	4.6	17.3	11.5
Pre-term	6.2	2.6	10.9
Low birthweight (up to 2500 grams)	5.7	2.0	11.1
Head circ. 32 cms or less	10.3	7.5	15.3
Length 47 cms or less	10.4	7.7	15.4
Special care	8.6	3.6	16.2
Breast feeding	69.9	71.7	62.2

*67 women who had episiotomy as well as laceration and are included in both groups.

**1888 of the women who had an intact perineum had had a Caesarean section.

TABLE A.17

Post-partum haemorrhage (PPH)

Factors	PPH (n = 1487) %	No PPH (n = 10214) %	
Primiparous	48.2	34.0	
Under 25 years	22.9	22.4	NS
Married	89.8	90.0	NS
Social class I, II	22.7	24.9	NS
Caucasian	88.2	86.4	NS
Asian	4.8	4.5	NS
Afro-Caribbean	4.1	3.2	NS
Under 160 cms tall	35.6	34.0	NS
Hypertension	13.2	8.4	
Ante-partum haemorrhage	6.0	2.3	
Induced labour	13.6	12.1	NS
Occipito-anterior	74.6	89.7	
Multiple pregnancy	3.5	1.1	
1st stage 6 hrs or more	35.5	22.1	
2nd stage 1 hr or more	51.5	26.6	
Forceps	22.9	19.2	
Elective section	18.8	4.8	
Emergency section	34.7	6.2	
Episiotomy	33.3	45.2	
Laceration	9.8	27.0	
Post-partum haemorrhage	–	–	
Epidural	59.2	38.0	
Pethidine	10.4	14.7	
Inhalation	24.3	44.6	
Tranquillisers	3.4	6.1	
Pudendal block	2.6	2.4	NS
Spinal block	1.7	1.3	NS
General anaesthetic	30.6	6.9	
No analgesia or anaesthesia	2.5	11.1	
Pre-term	10.1	6.4	
Low birthweight (up to 2500 grams)	9.5	6.1	
Head circ. 32 cms or less	11.7	11.2*	
Length 47 cms or less	13.0	11.2	
Special care	14.5	9.2	
Breast feeding	65.0	68.2	

*There was a statistical association between PPH and head circumference, measured as a continuous variable and using a T-test. The main feature was that women delivering babies with large heads were more likely to have a PPH.

TABLE A.18

Epidural anaesthesia

Factors	Epidural (n = 4766) %	No epidural (n = 6935) %	
Primiparous	48.8	26.8	
Under 25 years	23.2	21.9	NS
Married	89.9	89.9	NS
Social class I, II	26.5	24.5	
Caucasian	87.5	86.0	
Asian	4.2	4.7	NS
Afro-Caribbean	2.2	4.1	
Under 160 cms tall	35.2	33.5	NS
Hypertension	12.9	6.4	
Ante-partum haemorrhage	2.7	2.9	NS
Induced labour	19.8	7.1	
Occipito-anterior	82.3	91.5	
Multiple pregnancy	2.3	0.8	
1st stage 6 hrs or more	36.2	14.8	
2nd stage 1 hr or more	54.4	12.5	
Forceps	38.1	7.0	
Elective section	8.9	5.0	
Emergency section	13.7	7.1	
Episiotomy	56.7	34.8	
Laceration	13.4	32.7	
Post-partum haemorrhage	18.5	8.8	
Epidural	—	—	
Pethidine	6.6	19.4	
Inhalation	20.0	57.2	
Tranquillisers	2.1	8.2	
Pudendal block	0.7	3.6	
Spinal block	0.2	2.2	
General anaesthetic	6.4	12.3	
No analgesia or anaesthesia	N/A	N/A	
Pre-term	6.5	7.1	NS
Low birthweight (up to 2500 grams)	6.4	6.6*	
Head circ. 32 cms or less	10.0	12.1*	
Length 47 cms or less	10.6	12.0*	
Special care	10.7	9.3	
Breast feeding	66.8	68.5	NS

*There was a statistical association between epidural and birthweight measured as a continuous variable and using a T-test. The main feature was that the women delivering very large babies were more likely to have an epidural.

TABLE A.19

Pethidine

Factors	Pethidine (n = 1658) %	No pethidine (n = 10043) %	
Primiparous	52.2	33.0	
Under 25 years	31.8	20.9	
Married	86.6	90.5	
Social class I, II	18.9	25.6	
Caucasian	83.1	87.2	
Asian	5.9	4.3	
Afro-Caribbean	5.3	3.0	
Under 160 cms tall	35.3	34.0	NS
Hypertension	5.7	9.6	
Ante-partum haemorrhage	1.6	3.0	
Induced labour	13.6	12.1	NS
Occipito-anterior	87.2	91.6	
Multiple pregnancy	0.4	1.6	
1st stage 6 hrs or more	28.0	22.1	
2nd stage 1 hr or more	28.0	28.4	NS
Forceps	18.5	19.9	NS
Elective section	0.2	7.6	
Emergency section	5.9	10.4	
Episiotomy	52.1	42.3	
Laceration	26.1	24.6	NS
Post-partum haemorrhage	9.3	13.3	
Epidural	19.1	44.3	
Pethidine	–	–	
Inhalation	62.8	38.6	
Tranquillisers	24.7	2.6	
Pudendal block	4.6	2.1	
Spinal block	2.2	1.2	
General anaesthetic	3.9	10.9	
No analgesia or anaesthesia	N/A	N/A	
Pre-term	4.2	7.3	
Low birthweight (up to 2500 grams)	3.7	7.0	
Head circ. 32 cms or less	9.6	11.5	
Length 47 cms or less	10.7	11.5	NS
Special care	6.5	10.5	
Breast feeding	68.3	67.7	NS

TABLE A.20

Inhalation Analgesia

Factors	Inhalation (n = 4916) %	No inhalation (n = 6785) %	
Primiparous	34.0	37.0	
Under 25 years	24.2	21.1	
Married	89.3	90.4	
Social class I, II	22.7	26.1	
Caucasian	87.8	85.8	
Asian	4.3	4.7	NS
Afro-Caribbean	4.1	2.7	
Under 160 cms tall	32.7	35.3	
Hypertension	5.6	11.5	
Ante-partum haemorrhage	1.6	3.6	
Induced labour	8.6	15.0	
Occipito-anterior	92.9	84.1	
Multiple pregnancy	0.8	1.9	
1st stage 6 hrs or more	20.0	26.0	
2nd stage 1 hr or more	21.0	45.4	
Forceps	14.7	23.2	
Elective section	0.1	11.3	
Emergency section	3.3	14.5	
Episiotomy	44.2	43.3	NS
Laceration	33.7	18.4	
Post-partum haemorrhage	7.4	16.6	
Epidural	19.3	56.2	
Pethidine	21.2	9.1	
Inhalation	−	−	
Tranquillisers	8.0	4.2	
Pudendal block	3.5	1.6	
Spinal block	1.7	1.0	
General anaesthetic	2.4	15.3	
No analgesia or anaesthesia	N/A	N/A	
Pre-term	4.1	8.8	
Low birthweight (up to 2500 grams)	3.6	8.7	
Head circ. 32 cms or less	9.4	12.6	
Length 47 cms or less	9.3	12.9	
Special care	5.3	13.2	
Breast feeding	70.9	65.6	

TABLE A.21

Tranquillisers

Factors	Tranquillisers (n = 673) %	No tranquillisers (n = 11028) %	
Primiparous	48.7	35.0	
Under 25 years	28.7	22.1	
Married	89.2	90.0	NS
Social class I, II	21.1	24.8	
Caucasian	82.6	86.9	NS
Asian	4.0	4.6	NS
Afro-Caribbean	3.3	3.3	NS
Under 160 cms tall	33.6	34.3	NS
Hypertension	9.1	9.0	NS
Ante-partum haemorrhage	1.6	2.9	NS
Induced labour	13.7	12.2	NS
Occipito-anterior	90.6	87.6	
Multiple pregnancy	0.9	1.5	NS
1st stage 6 hrs or more	27.3	22.8	
2nd stage 1 hr or more	24.0	28.7	
Forceps	16.6	19.8	
Elective section	0.1	7.0	
Emergency section	6.1	10.0	
Episiotomy	57.2	42.9	
Laceration	19.8	25.2	
Post-partum haemorrhage	7.4	13.0	
Epidural	15.2	42.3	
Pethidine	60.8	11.3	
Inhalation	58.1	41.0	
Tranquillisers	—	—	
Pudendal block	5.5	2.7	
Spinal block	2.2	1.3	
General anaesthetic	4.2	10.2	
No analgesia or anaesthesia	N/A	N/A	
Pre-term	4.5	7.0	
Low birthweight (up to 2500 grams)	4.0	6.7	
Head circ. 32 cms or less	8.3	11.4	
Length 47 cms or less	10.7	11.5	NS
Special care	8.3	10.0	NS
Breast feeding	67.8	67.8	NS

TABLE A.22

Pudendal block

Factors	Pudendal block (n = 284) %	No pudendal block (n = 11417) %	
Primiparous	65.8	35.0	
Under 25 years	22.9	22.4	NS
Married	92.9	89.9	NS
Social class I, II	25.0	24.6	NS
Caucasian	91.9	86.5	
Asian	3.2	4.6	
Afro-Caribbean	1.4	3.4	
Under 160 cms tall	29.6	34.3	NS
Hypertension	9.2	9.0	NS
Ante-partum haemorrhage	1.8	2.8	NS
Induced labour	13.4	12.3	NS
Occipito-anterior	81.0	87.9	
Multiple pregnancy	2.1	1.4	NS
1st stage 6 hrs or more	27.0	23.0	
2nd stage 1 hr or more	52.3	27.7	
Forceps	79.6	18.2	
Elective section	−	6.7	
Emergency section	0.7	10.0	
Episiotomy	93.3	42.5	
Laceration	5.3	25.3	
Post-partum haemorrhage	13.7	12.7	NS
Epidural	12.3	41.4	
Pethidine	27.1	13.8	
Inhalation	60.9	41.5	
Tranquillisers	13.0	5.6	
Pudendal block	−	−	
Spinal block	2.1	1.3	NS
General anaesthetic	0.4	10.1	
No analgesia or anaesthesia	N/A	N/A	
Pre-term	5.6	6.9	NS
Low birthweight (up to 2500 grams)	6.7	6.6	NS
Head circ. 32 cms or less	11.3	11.3	NS
Length 47 cms or less	9.5	11.5	
Special care	8.8	9.9	NS
Breast feeding	71.8	67.7	NS

TABLE A.23

Factors	Spinal block		
	Spinal **(n = 160)** %	**No spinal** **(n = 11541)** %	
Primiparous	56.3	35.5	
Under 25 years	26.3	22.4	NS
Married	90.0	89.9	NS
Social class I, II	21.9	24.7	NS
Caucasian	87.5	86.6	NS
Asian	6.3	4.5	NS
Afro-Caribbean	2.5	3.3	NS
Under 160 cms tall	35.0	34.2	NS
Hypertension	6.9	9.0	NS
Ante-partum haemorrhage	1.3	2.8	NS
Induced labour	11.3	12.3	NS
Occipito-anterior	78.1	87.9	
Multiple pregnancy	0.6	1.5	NS
1st stage 6 hrs or more	26.2	23.0	
2nd stage 1 hr or more	61.6	27.9	
Forceps	65.0	19.0	
Elective section	—	6.7	
Emergency section	6.3	9.8	
Episiotomy	78.8	43.2	
Laceration	15.0	25.0	
Post-partum haemorrhage	16.3	12.7	NS
Epidural	6.3	41.2	
Pethidine	23.1	14.0	
Inhalation	51.9	41.9	
Tranquillisers	9.4	5.7	
Pudendal block	3.8	2.4	NS
Spinal block	—	—	
General anaesthetic	5.0	10.0	
No analgesia or anaesthesia	N/A	N/A	
Pre-term	5.0	6.9	NS
Low birthweight (up to 2500 grams)	5.0	6.6	NS
Head circ. 32 cms or less	8.8	11.3	NS
Length 47 cms or less	8.8	11.5	
Special care	8.1	9.9	NS
Breast feeding	70.0	67.8	NS

TABLE A.24

General anaesthetic*

Factors	General anaesthetic (n = 1158) %	No general anaesthetic (n = 10543) %	
Primiparous	40.3	35.3	
Under 25 years	18.2	22.9	
Married	90.9	89.8	NS
Social class I, II	25.1	24.6	NS
Caucasian	80.9	87.2	
Asian	6.6	4.3	
Afro-Caribbean	4.2	3.2	
Under 160 cms tall	44.0	33.1	
Hypertension	17.7	8.1	
Ante-partum haemorrhage	9.8	2.0	
Induced labour	10.1	12.5	
Occipito-anterior	66.9	90.2	
Multiple pregnancy	3.3	1.2	
1st stage 6 hrs or more	N/A	N/A	
2nd stage 1 hr or more	N/A	N/A	
Forceps	1.8	21.6	
Elective section	31.3	3.9	
Emergency section	65.0	3.7	
Episiotomy	3.2	48.1	
Laceration	0.5	27.5	
Post-partum haemorrhage	39.3	9.8	
Epidural	26.5	42.3	
Pethidine	5.5	15.1	
Inhalation	10.3	45.5	
Tranquillisers	2.4	6.1	
Pudendal block	0.1	2.7	
Spinal block	0.7	1.4	
General anaesthetic	—	—	
No analgesia or anaesthesia	N/A	N/A	
Pre-term	21.0	5.3	
Low birthweight (up to 2500 grams)	20.6	5.0	
Head circ. 32 cms or less	21.4	10.1	
Length 47 cms or less	23.1	10.1	
Special care	32.5	7.4	
Breast feeding	55.4	69.2	

*This includes general anaesthetic given for any procedure, although 98% were for sections.

We have also compared separately those women who had no analgesia or anaesthesia at all (Table A.25). This tended to occur in association with spontaneous onset of labour, short labour and normal delivery. Only 3.3% of those women having their first child had no analgesia or anaesthesia, compared with 13.7% of the multiparae.

Gestation at delivery (Table A.26). The comparison we give here is between pre-term associations, defined as deliveries before 37 weeks, and full-term deliveries. Pre-term deliveries were a little more frequent among primiparous and younger women. Women who had pre-term deliveries were much more likely (RR = 5.0) to have had an ante-partum haemorrhage and a little more likely to have had hypertension and an atypical fetal presentation. Both types of Caesarean section were closely associated with pre-term deliveries. Not surprisingly pre-term deliveries were also associated with smaller babies and admission to special care. Breast feeding was less common among pre-term deliveries.

Size of the baby (Tables A.27-A.29). Birthweight, head circumference and length of the baby were closely inter-related, as was gestation at delivery and admission to special care. Babies' size was also closely related to the characteristics of the mother. Smaller size was associated with primiparity, younger age, being unmarried, lower social class and being short in height. Race was highly associated with infant size. Both Asian and Afro-Caribbean women were more likely than white women to have a baby with a birthweight of 2500 grams or less (RR = 1.6 and 1.9 respectively). Similar magnitudes of differences according to race were also shown for the babies' head circumference and length. There was an association between small babies and maternal hypertension, ante-partum haemorrhage and atypical fetal presentation. Caesarean section of both types, but especially emergency, were more common in the delivery of smaller babies.

Special care admission (Table A.30) was closely associated with smaller infant size, pre-term delivery and Caesarean section. It was also associated to a lesser extent with primiparity, older maternal age and Asian and Afro-Caribbean race. Twins and triplets were much more likely to be admitted to special care.

Type of feeding on discharge (Table A.31) was associated much more closely with the characteristics of the mother and of the baby than with obstetric or anaesthetic factors. Primiparous, older and married women were more likely to breast feed. Social class I and II women and those of Afro-Caribbean race were much more likely to breast feed. Breast feeding was negatively associated with having a multiple pregnancy, a Caesarean section, a pre-term delivery, a smaller baby and a baby who was admitted to special care.

TABLE A.25

No analgesia or anaesthesia at all

Factors	No analgesia or anaesthetic (n = 1169) %	One or more type of analgesia/anaesthesia (n = 10532) %	
Primiparous	12.0	38.4	
Under 25 years	18.9	22.8	
Married	90.7	89.9	NS
Social class I, II	26.0	24.5	NS
Caucasian	86.9	86.6	NS
Asian	4.6	4.5	NS
Afro-Caribbean	3.9	3.2	NS
Under 160 cms tall	31.5	34.5	
Hypertension	3.5	9.6	
Ante-partum haemorrhage	1.5	2.9	
Induced labour	4.3	13.2	
Occipito-anterior	95.6	86.6	
Multiple pregnancy	0.3	1.6	
1st stage 6 hrs or more	8.8	24.1	
2nd stage 1 hr or more	5.6	31.5	
Forceps	0.6	21.8	
Elective section	N/A	N/A	
Emergency section	N/A	N/A	
Episiotomy	19.9	46.3	
Laceration	43.1	22.8	
Post-partum haemorrhage	3.2	13.8	
Epidural	N/A	N/A	
Pethidine	N/A	N/A	
Inhalation	N/A	N/A	
Tranquillisers	N/A	N/A	
Pudendal block	N/A	N/A	
Spinal block	N/A	N/A	
General anaesthetic	N/A	N/A	
No analgesia or anaesthesia	—	—	
Pre-term	4.6	7.1	
Low birthweight (up to 2500 grams)	4.3	6.8	
Head circ. 32 cms or less	12.7	11.1	
Length 47 cms or less	9.9	11.6	NS
Special care	4.9	10.4	
Breast feeding	70.5	67.5	

TABLE A.26

Gestation at delivery

Factors	Pre-term (n = 800) %	Term (n = 10901) %	
Primiparous	41.8	35.3	
Under 25 years	25.0	22.2	
Married	87.8	90.1	
Social class I, II	23.3	24.7	NS
Caucasian	85.0	86.7	NS
Asian	5.4	4.5	NS
Afro-Caribbean	4.0	3.3	NS
Under 160 cms tall	31.9	34.4	
Hypertension	17.5	8.4	
Ante-partum haemorrhage	11.0	2.2	
Induced labour	8.3	12.6	
Occipito-anterior	74.9	88.7	
Multiple pregnancy	9.4	0.9	
1st stage 6 hrs or more	19.7	23.2	
2nd stage 1 hr or more	23.1	28.7	
Forceps	14.4	20.1	
Elective section	10.4	6.3	
Emergency section	28.6	8.4	
Episiotomy	39.9	44.0	
Laceration	9.6	26.0	
Post-partum haemorrhage	18.8	12.3	
Epidural	38.9	40.9	NS
Pethidine	8.8	14.6	
Inhalation	25.1	43.3	
Tranquillisers	3.8	5.9	
Pudendal block	2.0	2.5	NS
Spinal block	1.0	1.4	NS
General anaesthetic	30.4	8.4	
No analgesia or anaesthesia	6.8	10.2	
Pre-term	–	–	
Low birthweight (up to 2500 grams)	60.3	2.6	
Head circ. 32 cms or less	53.1	8.4	
Length 47 cms or less	60.0	7.7	
Special care	72.9	5.3	
Breast feeding	54.9	68.8	

TABLE A.27

Birthweight

Factors	Up to 2500 grams (n = 767) %	2501-3600 grams (n = 7372) %	3601 grams or more (n = 3562) %	
Primiparous	43.9	38.2	29.0	
Under 25 years	23.1	23.5	20.2	
Married	86.4	89.0	92.7	
Social class I, II	19.6	23.7	27.7	
Caucasian	80.7	85.3	90.6	
Asian	6.8	5.4	2.2	
Afro-Caribbean	5.9	3.7	1.9	
Under 160 cms tall	37.3	37.9	25.9	
Hypertension	21.0	8.1	8.4	
Ante-partum haemorrhage	9.9	2.7	1.5	
Induced labour	10.6	11.5	14.3	
Occipito-anterior	72.2	89.1	88.3	
Multiple pregnancy	N/A	N/A	N/A	
1st stage 6 hrs or more	17.7	22.4	25.2	
2nd stage 1 hr or more	17.5	27.8	31.4	
Forceps	12.5	19.7	21.2	
Elective section	10.7	6.4	6.0	
Emergency section	30.4	7.8	9.4	
Episiotomy	37.9	43.5	45.4	
Laceration	7.6	25.1	28.0	
Post-partum haemorrhage	18.5	10.8	15.4	
Epidural	40.0	39.8	42.8	
Pethidine	8.0	15.0	13.7	
Inhalation	23.2	43.1	43.8	
Tranquillisers	3.5	5.8	6.1	
Pudendal block	2.5	2.3	2.6	NS
Spinal block	1.0	1.3	1.5	NS
General anaesthetic	31.2	8.4	8.3	
No analgesia or anaesthesia	6.5	10.4	9.8	
Pre-term	62.8	4.2	0.3	
Low birthweight (up to 2500 grams)	–	–	–	
Head circ. 32 cms or less	76.7	9.7	0.4	
Length 47 cms or less	65.8	10.6	1.3	
Special care	78.1	5.6	4.0	
Breast feeding	52.7	68.5	69.7	

TABLE A.28

Head circumference*

Factors

	Up to 32 cms (n = 1317) %	33-35 cms (n = 7853) %	Over 35 cms (n = 2459) %	
Primiparous	45.1	35.2	32.9	
Under 25 years	27.8	22.5	19.6	
Married	86.1	89.7	92.6	
Social class I, II	19.6	24.6	27.3	
Caucasian	79.1	86.8	91.0	
Asian	8.0	4.6	2.6	
Afro-Caribbean	6.5	3.4	1.5	
Under 160 cms tall	41.8	35.3	26.6	
Hypertension	12.8	8.4	9.0	
Ante-partum haemorrhage	6.8	2.4	1.8	
Induced labour	9.8	11.3	16.9	
Occipito-anterior	82.8	89.0	86.5	
Multiple pregnancy	6.5	1.0	0.2	
1st stage 6 hrs or more	17.0	22.1	25.4	
2nd stage 1 hr or more	21.9	26.6	38.2	
Forceps	15.0	19.4	23.1	
Elective section	5.9	5.9	9.0	
Emergency section	18.2	7.7	11.9	
Episiotomy	40.1	43.9	45.1	
Laceration	16.5	26.7	24.0	
Post-partum haemorrhage	13.2	11.2	17.3	
Epidural	36.2	39.3	47.9	
Pethidine	12.1	15.2	12.1	NS
Inhalation	34.9	44.1	39.4	
Tranquillisers	4.3	6.2	5.2	
Pudendal block	2.4	2.5	2.3	NS
Spinal block	1.1	1.3	1.7	NS
General anaesthetic	18.8	7.9	11.1	
No analgesia or anaesthesia	11.2	10.5	7.8	
Pre-term	36.4	3.6	0.9	
Low birthweight (up to 2500 grams)	44.6	2.1	0.1	
Head circ. 32 cms or less	–	–	–	
Length 47 cms or less	35.1	6.4	1.9	
Special care	43.0	5.7	5.0	
Breast feeding	61.5	68.4	69.8	

*Those 72 cases where head circumference was not recorded are excluded from this Table.

TABLE A.29

Length of baby*

Factors

	Up to 47 cms (n = 1336) %	48-52 cms (n = 6356) %	Over 52 cms (n = 3809) %	
Primiparous	39.7	35.5	35.4	
Under 25 years	24.3	23.2	20.6	
Married	87.3	89.6	91.3	
Social class I, II	21.9	24.3	25.9	
Caucasian	82.4	86.1	89.9	
Asian	6.5	4.9	3.3	
Afro-Caribbean	5.3	3.5	2.2	
Under 160 cms tall	39.1	36.1	29.3	
Hypertension	14.7	7.9	8.6	
Ante-partum haemorrhage	5.8	2.7	1.9	
Induced labour	10.6	11.5	14.2	
Occipito-anterior	81.4	89.1	88.5	
Multiple pregnancy	6.5	1.0	0.2	
1st stage 6 hrs or more	19.3	21.3	25.0	
2nd stage 1 hr or more	22.0	27.3	32.5	
Forceps	14.5	19.1	22.9	
Elective section	10.2	6.7	4.8	
Emergency section	18.0	7.9	8.8	
Episiotomy	40.0	43.7	45.4	
Laceration	16.8	25.5	27.5	
Post-partum haemorrhage	14.5	11.2	14.3	
Epidural	37.6	39.5	44.1	
Pethidine	13.2	15.1	13.4	
Inhalation	34.3	42.7	44.8	
Tranquillisers	5.4	6.1	5.4	NS
Pudendal block	2.0	2.2	3.1	
Spinal block	1.0	1.1	1.8	
General anaesthetic	20.0	8.7	7.0	
No analgesia or anaesthesia	8.7	10.4	9.8	NS
Pre-term	31.8	4.2	0.9	
Low birthweight (up to 2500 grams)	37.8	2.2	0.3	
Head circ. 32 cms or less	42.5	9.3	2.7	
Length 47 cms or less	—	—	—	
Special care	38.0	6.1	4.3	
Breast feeding	62.7	67.8	70.5	

* Those 200 cases where length was not recorded are excluded from the Table.

TABLE A.30

Admission of baby to special care (SCBU)

Factors	Special care (n = 1156) %	No SCBU (n = 10545) %	
Primiparous	42.9	35.0	
Under 25 years	22.1	22.5*	
Married	88.6	90.1	NS
Social class I, II	22.1	24.9	NS
Caucasian	83.5	87.0	
Asian	5.1	4.5	
Afro-Caribbean	3.7	3.3	
Under 160 cms tall	33.3	34.3*	
Hypertension	19.2	7.9	
Ante-partum haemorrhage	8.0	2.2	
Induced labour	15.8	11.9	
Occipito-anterior	75.3	89.1	
Multiple pregnancy	8.3	0.7	
1st stage 6 hrs or more	23.8	23.0	NS
2nd stage 1 hr or more	24.9	29.1	
Forceps	15.6	20.1	
Elective section	13.4	5.8	
Emergency section	29.5	7.6	
Episiotomy	38.1	44.3	
Laceration	9.2	26.6	
Post-partum haemorrhage	18.7	12.1	
Epidural	44.0	40.4	
Pethidine	9.3	14.7	
Inhalation	22.5	44.2	
Tranquillisers	4.8	5.9	NS
Pudendal block	2.2	2.5	NS
Spinal block	1.1	1.4	NS
General anaesthetic	32.5	7.4	
No analgesia or anaesthesia	4.9	10.5	
Pre-term	50.4	2.1	
Low birthweight (up to 2500 grams)	51.8	1.6	
Head circ. 32 cms or less	49.0	7.1	
Length 47 cms or less	43.9	7.9	
Special care	–	–	
Breast feeding	54.1	69.3	

*There were statistical associations between SCBU and maternal age and height measured as a continuous variable using a T-test. The main features were that older mothers and shorter mothers were more likely to have a baby who was admitted to SCBU.

TABLE A.31

Type of feeding on discharge

Factors	Breast* (n = 7937) %	Artificial (n = 3764) %	
Primiparous	38.6	29.7	
Under 25 years	19.1	29.5	
Married	91.3	87.1	
Social class I, II	30.4	12.5	
Caucasian	85.5	88.2	
Asian	4.2	5.3	
Afro-Caribbean	4.3	1.2	
Under 160 cms tall	31.6	39.7	
Hypertension	8.5	10.1	
Ante-partum haemorrhage	2.5	3.5	
Induced labour	11.7	13.5	
Occipito-anterior	88.5	86.7	
Multiple pregnancy	1.0	2.4	
1st stage 6 hrs or more	23.7	21.7	NS
2nd stage 1 hr or more	28.8	27.4	NS
Forceps	20.2	18.5	
Elective section	5.9	8.0	
Emergency section	8.6	12.3	
Episiotomy	45.0	40.9	
Laceration	26.2	21.9	
Post-partum haemorrhage	12.2	13.8	
Epidural	40.1	42.0	NS
Pethidine	14.3	13.9	NS
Inhalation	43.9	38.0	
Tranquillisers	5.7	5.8	NS
Pudendal block	2.6	2.1	NS
Spinal block	1.7	1.3	NS
General anaesthetic	8.1	13.7	
No analgesia or anaesthesia	10.4	9.2	
Pre-term	5.5	9.6	
Low birthweight (up to 2500 grams)	5.1	9.6	
Head circ. 32 cms or less	10.2	13.5	
Length 47 cms or less	10.6	13.2	
Special care	7.9	14.1	
Breast feeding	–	–	

*238 women who were breast feeding with artificial supplements are included here as breast.

Conclusions

To anyone who knows only a litle about obstetrics it will immediately be obvious that many of the associations we have described are indirect ones. We have not generally attempted in this Appendix to assess which of the associations are primary and which are indirect although some are obvious. Our main intention was to demonstrate that a complex inter-relationship exists between many of the maternal, obstetric and anaesthetic characteristics, by showing for reference purposes the exact nature of all these associations.

Coventry University

Printed in the UK for HMSO
Dd 294076 C 10/91